THE HISTORY OF REGIONAL MEDICAL PROGRAMS

The Life and Death of a Small Initiative of the Great Society

Stephen P. Strickland

University Press of America
Lanham • New York • Oxford

Copyright © 2000 by
University Press of America,® Inc.

4720 Boston Way
Lanham, Maryland 20706

12 Hid's Copse Rd.
Cumnor Hill, Oxford OX2 9JJ

Library of Congress Cataloging-in-Publication Data

Strickland, Stephen P. (Stephen Parks)
The history of regional medical programs : the life and death
of a small initiative of the Great Society / Stephen P. Strickland.
p.   cm.
Includes bibiographical references and index.
1.   Regional medical programs—United States—History—20th century.
2.   Social legislation—United States—History—20th century.
3. Medical policy—United States—History—20th century. I. Title
RA412.2.S77 2000   362.1'0973'09045—dc21   00—044330 CIP

ISBN 0-7618-1775-1 (cloth: alk. ppr)

To

Donald A. B. Lindberg, M. D.

Pioneer in medical communications,
Steady and creative leader of institutions

and

Mary M. Lindberg

Loyal friend to many,
Epitome of grace and caring

Contents

The History of Regional Medical Programs

Foreword

President Lyndon B. Johnson's plans for a "Great Society," and the array of programs he initiated in order to achieve it, have been reviewed by scores of scholars and analysts over the past thirty-five years. Some of these are clearly partisan or doctrinaire. Others seem quite objective but written for accountants. The more sweeping assessments may have been undertaken too soon.

It would be hard to argue that millions of Americans in the year 2000 are interested in any of this, even if Medicare pays their hospital bills or their children learned to read in a Head Start program. But the thoughtful recording of history can be of great value to those who care about the future, especially those concerned with charting the future, and the true lessons of history are in the details. Stephen Strickland's latest book, like his earlier ones, provides essential details in an engaging fashion about a remarkable enterprise. Here his subject is Regional Medical Programs, begun in 1965 by President Johnson after he received the report of his Commission on Heart Disease, Cancer and Stroke that was chaired by the famous heart surgeon, Dr. Michael DeBakey. The strong recommendations of the commission were watered down by Congress after heavy pressure from the American Medical Association. The program was terminated a decade later by President Richard Nixon and a reluctant, still predominantly Democratic Congress.

Regional Medical Programs' purpose was to put the latest advances in medical treatment – beginning with those for heart disease, cancer and stroke – at the disposal of physicians throughout the country, and so bring such advances to hundreds of communities and thousands of people who otherwise would be denied them. The purpose and the funds came from the top, but otherwise RMPs were organized locally, in states or metropolitan areas. They were implemented principally by health professionals based in a variety of institutions, particularly medical schools, and overseen by volunteer advisory boards that included lay citizens. In short, Regional Medical Programs were a typical American venture.

Much was accomplished in the course of the ten-year effort. Some relationships and structures erected under RMP's aegis did indeed serve as vehicles for the application of significant medical advances, especially in the prevention and treatment of cardiovascular disease. Dr. Strickland identifies other good particular results, and some nebulous ones, produced by the RMP initiative before it was overtaken by events on the big screen.

Emergency medical services were first created in some areas by RMPs. Medical staffs of many small hospitals were systematically linked to those of large teaching hospitals. Hundreds of coronary care nurses and technicians were trained. Two medical schools were established. The application of computers to medical diagnosis and rapid transfer of information was given a significant boost, as Dr. Donald Lindberg, Director of the National Library of Medicine will attest and as his institution makes manifest in thousands of life-enhancing instances every day. An estimated 1.5 million heart, cancer and stroke patients did receive up-to-date treatment through RMPs in a ten-year span.

Now another quarter-century has passed, and the author has used this distance, as well as dozens of contemporary sources, to capture the full picture and assess the value of the effort. In his fine, short history we can see both trees and forest. If we like, we can tally up the dollars spent and come to our own judgments about worth. What we cannot miss, in Dr. Strickland's account, is the deeply caring spirit that motivated the policy makers who conceived, and the great civic energy of the professional and citizen practitioner who gave life to, Regional Medical Programs.

Philip R. Lee, M.D.
Professor Emeritus and Senior Advisor
Institute of Health Policy Studies
School of Medicine
University of California, San Francisco

Introduction

In early February 1994 Mary Woodard Lasker died, leaving one of the most extraordinary legacies in influencing public policy and national health programs of any private citizen in American history. Possessed of enormous intelligence, moderate wealth, an array of friends in key places, relentless energy and focused purpose, Mrs. Lasker saw many of her ambitions realized. With her friend and partner in policy-shaping, Florence Stephenson Mahoney, she worked for the creation of the National Institutes of Health in the 1940's; helped build a solid constituency for increasing funds for NIH beginning in the 1950's; and worked for the passage of Medicare and other Great Society programs in the 1960's. In 1970, Mrs. Lasker forged one of the most unusual alliances in American politics, that between President Richard Nixon and Senator Edward Kennedy, persuading them to launch a new national "war on cancer."

Mary Lasker and her friend and ally Dr. Michael DeBakey were instrumental in conceptualizing and organizing several plans to help President Lyndon Johnson realize his objective of reducing the deadly impact of heart disease, cancer and stroke. A central component of the early strategy was a system of Regional Medical Programs, the original blueprint of which took only a year to formulate and ten months to legislate. Unfortunately for those who though it was a good idea the program took several years to implement. If Mike DeBakey was the "Father" of Regional Medical Programs, Mary Lasker was the "Godmother." Florence Mahoney, who served on the recommending commission, was one of the facilitators of the new initiative.

Thirty-five years have passed since Regional Medical Programs were officially launched. With the prominent exceptions of Dr. DeBakey, who is still going strong at 90 and Mrs. Mahoney, who in 1999 began her second century, many of the great political figures of that period are gone. But aside from the personalities, much of the political landscape looks the same.

In early 1994 President Clinton was surprised when the American Medical Association, after endorsing his overall plan for national health care, withdrew its support.   Thirty years earlier, President Johnson was surprised when the AMA, after tacitly joining in the effort to create a program to reduce heart disease, cancer and stroke, withdrew its representative on the relevant national commission just weeks before its report was released, then organized a concerted, hyperbolic and very bitter campaign against it.

The justification for wholesale reform of the health care system, said President Clinton, lay in the fact that the country was faced with a health care crisis.   That phrase had first been used in a presidential address in, 1971, by President Nixon.   Twenty years later, President Clinton and his principal health policy partner, First Lady Hillary Rodham Clinton, proposed a new plan whereby the financing would be on a national basis, but many of the decisions about provision of care would be made locally, by individuals and local providers. They indicated that states ought to have broad oversight authority, were to be central actors in the overall plan.   Implicitly the proposal recognized the now established pattern of regional concentrations of health care providers and other resources.

It was in 1964 that President Johnson and his Commission of Heart Disease, Cancer and Stroke identified the need to build networks of regional resources.   The Congress and subsequently the medical community agreed, though they insisted that the regional arrangements must be pulled together cooperatively, collegially, voluntarily.

The story that follows attempts to chronicle the history of the Heart Disease, Cancer and Stroke Amendments of 1965, subsequently known as Regional Medical Programs.   It is a history of an enterprise fraught with problems, but energized by the will, skill and imagination of scores of public officials and citizens who, over the decade of the program's formal existence, bent every effort to insure that realization of fundamental purpose: putting the best, most advanced medical knowledge within the reach of the greatest number of citizens.

The underlying problem that stood in the way of realization of the RMP purpose has not been much altered in the past thirty-five years.   That obstacle, in Irving Lewis' phrase, is "the excessively pluralistic character of American society," especially including those elements that aggregate into what is called the health care system. Another sometime architect and long-time observer of federal health programs, Dr. William Kissick, puts it thus: " In the American health care system, E. Pluribus Unum means a lot of pluribus and a dash of unum."

Whether there are in the history of Regional Medical Programs broad, fundamental or even particular lessons for the reform of American health care must be left to others to decide. But the RMP story does illustrate again certain truths about public policy and national enterprises: They cannot fully succeed without consistency of purpose and steadiness in implementation and funding.

There is another aspect to the story of Regional Medical Programs that reveals itself to a historian and analyst of national health policy. It is that a changing context, including the identification of new national needs or new recognition of old systemic flaws, can change thoughtful judgments about what constitutes success or failure. The good that is done through collaborative human efforts, like that of individuals, should not be interred with their bones. In my judgments, Regional Medical Programs did much good.

It takes a community of friends and colleagues to build a book. I am blessed, once more, with a sizable, knowledgeable and loyal group of such friends and colleagues. Only a few of them are specified below, but all of them I thank most sincerely for their contributions to this volume, which has been several years in the making. Many of these persons are named in the text, for they were involved in the creation, implementation or oversight of Regional Medical Programs. In fundamental ways, this is their story.

The leaders and staff of the National Library of Medicine, as well as that institution's archives, have been the main support system for this effort. I inhabited the History of Medicine Division for many months over a couple of years, and am grateful to Dr. Philip Teigen, then acting director of the division, and to Monique Young, its principal secretary, for many acts of assistance and kindness. Dr. Alexa

McCray, Director of the Lister Hill National Center for Biomedical Communications, created electronic linkages for the Library's traditional archival materials on Regional Medical Programs, and my early and on-going work on the topic, with a braoder public. She was generous with her time and technical knowledge, and with her secretary, the wonderful and impeccable Jackie Duley, who made the final version of this manuscript acceptable to the publisher. It is a gratifying wonder to this late-comer to the computer age to know that an instantly accessible information base, in addition to the printed page, can help relay the history of Regional Medical Programs.

The first and continuous inspiration for my final (I trust) examination of national health policies and programs is the truly distinguished Director of the National Library of Medicine, Dr. Donald A. B. Lindberg. His early experience in medical and biomedical communications, in part within the framework of the Missouri Regional Medical Program, was an important factor in his ultimately coming to Bethesda to lead the Library, which he has done in brilliant, solid fashion since 1984.

I am grateful to my colleagues of the National Peace Foundation who filled gaps during my regular absences from our offices in Washington in order to be in Bethesda, and my occasional additional absences in order to interview some of those who helped build RMPs in Seatle, Columbia, Missouri, Philadelphia, New York, New Haven, Cleveland, Atlanta, Birmingham, North Carolina and elsewhere. Glen Morin of our Foundation staff served as an able resercher and diligent computerist in the early and later months of this long project, and I am keenly appreciative of his help. Kathleen Lansing, Vice President of the Foundation, kept the work moving steadily along with or without me.

There are three long-time friends and mentors whom I have called upon, over three decades, for general counsel about and specific assistance with my several health policy and history projects including this one. They are: Dr. John F. Sherman, Dr. S. Richardson Hill, and Dr. Philip R. Lee, all three deeply knowledgeable and eminently wise, distinguished in their human goodness as well as their professional service and achievements. My indebtedness to them is profound.

I trust that the contributions of all are made clear by these words and the detail of the book's text. I am fully aware that any errors of omission or commission are mine alone.

Stephen P. Strickland, Ph.D.
Washington, DC
April, 2000

Chapter 1

The President's Commission

President Lyndon Johnson was both a "people person" and a program person. Specifically and emphatically, he believed that programs like those his hero Franklin D. Roosevelt had created and like those he himself was getting enacted, really did help real people. He believed, moreover, that federal programs -- whether centrally run (e.g. Social Security) or centrally funded but state-directed (e.g., Hill-Burton hospital construction) -- were sometimes the only way to insure that large numbers of people in need were helped.

To anyone who knew the President's personal and political history it was no surprise that more federal health, education and welfare laws were added to the books during his administration than during any other. His last Secretary of Health, Education and Welfare, Wilbur Cohen, proudly reported to his retiring boss in December 1968 that, in the five years of his presidency, 102 laws in these areas, including "sixty-two landmark enactments," had been enacted.[1] The statutory and programmatic landmarks in the health arena included: Medicare and Medicaid, four health manpower acts, four clean air acts, three extensions of the Hill-Burton Hospital Construction Act of 1948, the Partnership for Health Acts of 1966 and 1967, four Economic Opportunity Acts with their neighborhood health provisions, and the "Heart Disease, Cancer and Stroke Act of 1965."[2]

President Johnson felt the need for studies, for expert assessments of problems and issues, even when he had his own instincts about them. LBJ probably appointed more commissions to deal with more subjects than any other president in American history. He took their reports seriously and tried to implement their recommendations. He was especially inclined to ask for and accept advice from persons he knew or, next best, from persons whom his friends personally knew and assured him were the leading experts.

Less than two months after he assumed the presidency, Lyndon Johnson presented his Health Message to Congress, in January 1964. In it he reported that he was establishing a commission on heart disease, cancer and strokes to reduce the incidents of these three diseases which, he stated, "now afflict 15 million Americans -- two-thirds of all Americans now living will ultimately suffer or die from one of them."[3] Not that the federal government was not already working on the problem; the Public Health Service, the President noted, was already spending a quarter of a billion dollars annually to find ways to combat these diseases, and other public and private organizations were also involved. Further, "the flow of new discoveries, new drugs, new techniques" were impressive and hopeful. However, "much remains to be learned." Meanwhile, "the American people are not receiving the full benefits of what medical research has already accomplished."[4]

There was no blame cast. In part, the President said, the problem had to do with shortages of professional health workers and medical facilities. "It is also partly due to the public's lack of awareness of recent developments and techniques of prevention and treatment." The new commission would be asked how to bridge the gaps, including both those having to do with the need for new knowledge and "more complete utilization of the medical knowledge we already have."[5]

In fact, the concrete idea of a new government-sponsored look at the treatment of heart disease and cancer had appeared in the Democratic Party's 1960 platform. Dr. Michael DeBakey had been chairman of an ad hoc committee advising the platform committee on health matters. A friend of his -- and of the man who turned out to be the Party's nominee, Senator John F. Kennedy -- Mrs. Mary Lasker, had been urging such a proposal for some time.[6]

Soon after his election President Kennedy asked for a study. The group that worked on it included Dr. DeBakey. Unfortunately, the resulting report was to be presented to the President on the day of the Bay of Pigs invasion. For that obvious reason and, according to journalist Elizabeth Drew, because the report "was so badly done that it was a bit of disaster in its own right," the report was never officially presented, accepted or acted upon.[7] "The Lasker forces pushed for another commission," wrote Drew, one that would add stroke to the study mandate, presumably because the President's father had suffered a stroke. President Kennedy was said to be considering a new commission when he was assassinated. But Mary Lasker, Mike DeBakey and their friends-in-arms never give up.[8]

It was about the first of March 1964 that Dr. DeBakey received a call from the White House. The President wanted to know whether Dr. DeBakey would be willing to chair a blue-ribbon commission to advise him on measures to reduce the impact of the dread diseases. Dr. DeBakey accepted. On March 7th, the President announced the names of the other members of the Commission which Dr. DeBakey would chair. On April 17, the President invited the Commission to come to the White House for its first meeting. As DeBakey noted, Lyndon Johnson had "a very effective way of discussing matters with individuals or with groups and persuading them, so to speak, to work for him. He has a very effective way of inspiring and stimulating people."[9]

The President said to his Commission,

Health is something that we treasure in this house where you are gathered this morning, and I know it is treasured in every house throughout our land and around the world.

The work that you have begun today is work in which I have the keenest and greatest and the most personal interest. You are here to begin mapping an attack by this nation upon the three great killers, the three great cripplers -- heart, cancer and stroke disease.....

I want us to put our great resources -- and they are unlimited -- to work to overcome this... Because of the work that you will do, I believe that we will... I am firmly convinced that the accumulated brains and determination of this commission and of the scientific community for the world will, before the end of this decade, come forward with some answers and cures that we need so very much. When this occurs -- not if, but when, and I emphasize when -- we will face a new challenge and that will be what to do within our economy to adjust ourselves to a life-span and a workspan for the average man or woman of 100 years.[10]

The President acknowledged that the task he laid on the Commission was a heavy one, but felt sure that "their talents and their energies and their imagination" would get the job done. And a successful job would be a proud legacy.

In my judgment there is nothing that you will ever do that will keep your name glorified longer, and that will make your descendants prouder than this unselfish task that you have undertaken to get rid of the causes of heart disease and cancer and stroke in this land and around the world.

I am here to say to you that while we are interested in the food stamp plan, we are interested in Medicare for the aged under social security, we are interested in the Civil Rights Bill that we consider most essential to our leadership in this country and in the world, we are interested in the Pay Bill that will keep our good civil servants here, we are interested in the Immigration Bill that will permit families to join each other, and we are interested in the Poverty Bill that will take our boys out of the pool halls and out of the slums and out of the juvenile delinquency centers of the nation -- we are interested in all these things -- there is nothing that really offers more and greater hope to all humanity and to preserving humanity than the challenge and the task you have undertaken.

There was only one more thing: Would the Commission be good enough to begin its comprehensive survey and then offer its specific recommendations before the end of the year, so that he could propose appropriate legislation to the next Congress as soon as it convened in January 1965?

Those whom President Johnson asked to help him decide what should be done included many persons he knew. These included Mrs. Harry Truman, the widow of the President;*[13] his own heart doctor, Dr. J. Willis Hurst of Emory University; and a long-time, friend Mrs. Florence Mahoney, who with Mary Lasker had organized and helped to lead the "Health Syndicate," the self-appointed, unpaid, and highly effective citizens' lobby for better health care and more money for biomedical research.[14] Also on the commission were other important members of the medical research lobby, including Emerson Foote, one of Albert Lasker's early proteges; Dr. Sydney Farber of the Children's Cancer Hospital in Boston; Dr. Howard Rusk, a pioneer in rehabilitation medicine; Dr. Irving Wright, Chairman, National Advisory Heart Council; General Alfred Gruenther of the American Red Cross. Other distinguished public figures named were Dr. Phillip Handler, soon to become President of the National Academy of Sciences; Barry Bingham, publisher of the Louisville Courier; General David Sarnoff, founder and president of NBC; and Marion Folsom who had served in the Eisenhower Administration as Secretary of Health, Education and Welfare.[15]

Beyond the core group of commission members allied with the Lasker consortium, the reach of the President was relatively wide. The composition of the commission was diverse in a variety of ways. There were, of course, many physicians, among them a representative of the American Medical Association, Dr. Hugh H. Hussy, Director of AMA's Division of Scientific Activities. There were several women members, including a black physician whose specialty was oncology, Dr. Jane Wright of the New York University School of Medicine.

The physicians contingent included several medical school department chairmen: Dr. DeBakey himself; Dr. Hurst who chaired Emory's Department of Internal Medicine, Dr. John Meyer who chaired Penn State University College of Medicine's Department of Uterology, Dr. E. M. Pepper who chaired the Department of Anesthesiology of Columbia's College of Physicians and Surgeons; and Dr. Howard Rusk who chaired New York University Medical Center's Department of Physical Medicine Rehabilitation.

There were two former medical school deans, Dr. Edward W. Dempsey, earlier Dean of the School of Medicine at Washington University and Dr. Marion S. Fay, former President and Dean of the Women's Medical College of Pennsylvania. There was, however, no representative per se of the medical schools. For example, no one represented the Association of American Medical Colleges to which all medical schools in the country belong. Yet the Commission's interest in and concern about the health of medical schools, as well as the health of the people of the country, was manifest. Not only did the Commission place medical schools at the center of its three principal recommendations, but it was one of the first public bodies to recommend a program of direct federal subsidy of medical education.

The Commission was staffed principally by key professionals in the Public Health Service, even though the staff director, Dr. Abraham Lilienfeld, came to the enterprise from the Johns Hopkins University

School of Hygiene and Public Health. Also on staff was a brilliant writer, Marcus Rosenbloom, whose special talent was translating often complicated technical jargon into language comprehensible to laymen, including congressmen and presidents.

Dr. DeBakey named as "principal consultant" the equally brilliant legislative and political strategist Mike Gorman, who, as Executive Director of the National Committee Against Mental Illness, was Mary Lasker's point man in Washington. Bill Kissick says that Gorman served as a de facto co-chair and coordinator, making sure that Dr. DeBakey had all the information and support he needed on a daily basis and that work proceeded at a pace and in directions Mrs. Lasker and the President would approve of.

The Commission appointed subcommittees on the three principal diseases, and also on facilities, training, and communications.

In all, the Commission possessed an extraordinary aggregate knowledge and experience which, along with the President's direct, personal and highly public mandate, proved extremely useful. Its combined network of professional contacts was equally important; other major health proposals were in development, including those on Medicare and Medicaid, which had the attention of major constituencies who needed to be consulted about heart disease, cancer and stroke.

The Commission organized quickly, in part because of the Public Health Service staff. It promptly asked agencies, institutions, associations and any other entity concerned with the relevant diseases to provide any information they had already gathered. It set up a series of hearings at which expert witnesses from the widest possible range of interests, both public and private, presented their views. And it turned over to the subcommittee chairs, who were to make up an executive committee of the Commission, the job of sorting through information and relating it to their principal concerns. The Commission asked the Chairman of the Council of Economic Advisors to do a detailed analysis of the economic costs of the diseases. It established liaisons with the American Heart Association, the American Cancer Society, and key state and local health agencies.

In six months, it held forty-five meetings, heard from more than 165 experts, and obtained more than 7,500 pages of testimony which added up to "many millions of words." The Commission as a whole met six times between April and December, several of the meetings being days' and nights' length. The executive committee held ten meetings.[16]

The report was indeed completed in time for presentation to the President in December 1964. There was, of course, a direct, oral presentation to the President. The printed report was contained in about 80 pages and included 35 specific recommendations, most dealing with heart, cancer and stroke, but others dealing with related health problems, including health resources and facilities and, in some cases, the reorganization of existing programs.*[17] Beyond the 35 substantive recommendations, the Commission also recommended an entire reorganization of the Department of Health, Education and Welfare.[18]

In short, there were two categories of recommendations, one set constituting "the frontal assaults on problems related the conquest of heart disease, cancer and stroke."[19] A second set was "designed to strengthen the total national resource for advancing scientific knowledge and providing medical services." The "frontal assault" recommendations — "the innovative thrust of the report" -- added up to "the establishment of a national network of regional centers, local diagnostic and treatment stations, and medical complexes designed to unite the worlds of scientific research, medical education and medical care."[20]

From the first, the Commission acknowledged the central, essential, indeed paramount role of doctors in the overall enterprise. "The first line of defense for our people's health is manned by private practitioners. The advance in biomedical research is led by individual investigators..." and "individual freedom is the cornerstone of the health structure."[21] But the goal was also clear: fusing the worlds of science and practice, developing creative partnerships among all health resources, and putting the federal government in position to "stimulate and support the upwardthrust of national health."[22]

There were reassurances, however, to any who might be concerned about a significantly expanded federal role. "The system is not designed to duplicate existing resources but to strengthen them. The purpose of the entire system is to assist the doctor in practice and the care of his patient who is suffering from heart disease, cancer or stroke. It will make available to every doctor in the country the newest most effective diagnostic methods and the most promising methods of treatment. It will, in effect, make available to every private doctor and every community hospital to a national -- indeed worldwide -- network transmitting the newest and best in health service."[23]

Recommendation #1 was "the establishment of a national network of Regional Heart Disease, Cancer and Stroke Centers for clinical investigation, teaching and patient care, in universities, hospital and research institutes and other institutions across the country."[24] The Commission thought that the country needed 25 such centers for heart disease, 20 for cancer, and 15 for stroke, to be established over a five-year period. It would cost about $850 million over that time span. The details for the organization and development of such centers was to be worked by an Advisory Committee to the Public Health Service which would report to the Surgeon General.[25]

The Commission noted that: "Centers already exist, particularly in cancer, which can serve as a nucleus for some of these regional centers." But: "Investments in potential sites with be necessary in places where the nucleus for these facilities does not exist."[26] The centers would be strongly oriented toward clinical investigation and fundamental research. They would conduct training programs for personnel staff in diagnostic and treatment stations and would also serve a teaching function for the medical community of the region.

As regards existing federal efforts in the field, the Commission noted that the U.S. Vocational Rehabilitation Administration already ran five rehabilitation centers around the country and suggested doubling the number of them. And it pointed to the NIH Clinical Center's program of clinical research units in various parts of the country and indicated the desire to build on those.

As a complement to the regional centers, the Commission's second recommendation was the establishment of "a national network of diagnostic and treatment stations in communities across the nation."[27] It specifically foresaw within a five-year period 150 such stations being established for heart disease, 200 for cancer, 100 for stroke and 100 for rehabilitation. The construction funds should come from the federal government but staffing and operating costs were to be borne in part by local resources. It envisioned that each station could become self-supporting within a 10-15 year period. The overall cost would be about $480 million.[28]

The third recommendation seemed to constitute the spoke in the wheel. It would create "broad and flexible program of grant support... to stimulate formation of medical complexes whereby university medical schools, hospitals and other health care and research agencies and institutions work in concert."[29] $250 million was recommended so that over five years, some 30 medical centers could transform themselves into "medical complexes serving a large community hospital, metropolitan area or region."[30]

This recommendation turned out to be the cause of greatest controversy as the report was digested, responded to, and addressed a few months later by Congress and the affected community. The Commission "envisioned" that approximately 10 medical centers would receive such grants in the first year -- the average grant being $2.5 million -- followed by five additional centers around the country for the next four years.[31]

As a supplement, because more "centers of excellence" were needed, the Commission recommended a program of development grants to medical schools "to improve their total capability for both academic and research programs."[32] It had in mind, the Commission noted, existing funds for institutional development administered by the National Science Foundation, with which the new government program should be carefully coordinated. The purpose, said the Commission, was to raise a number of medical institutions of demonstrated potential to a level of excellence comparable to the few existing outstanding medical centers of the nation. The price tag for this component was only $40 million over a five year period.[33]

The Commission acknowledged the central roles of the National Heart Institute and the National Cancer Institute in waging the battle against those dread diseases. To balance out the organizational and categorical disease enterprise, its fifth recommendation was the establishment of a National Stroke Program. This would be developed with the advice of a joint subcommittee for cerebrovascular diseases of the National Advisory of Heart Council and the National Advisory of the Neurological Diseases and Blindness Council.[34]

Beyond the first five recommendations, there were thirty others which in the commission's judgment would also move the nation toward the conquest of heart disease, cancer and stroke. They had to do with community programs, with state programs, with continuing education, with further support for the already burgeoning biomedical science enterprise centered in the National Institutes of Health.

As indicated, there were in the introduction to the Commission's report specific words of reassurance to private medical doctors and to community hospitals. There was praise for the private health associations, including those dealing with cancer and heart and other major diseases. But it was the federal health establishment -- federal institutions and programs — that should have been very much reassured by a commission operating under the President's personal and direct mandate and with broad powers to recommend to him what to recommend to the Congress.

The Commission urged cooperation with the National Science Foundation, some of whose programs it praised;[35] it recommended that the Veterans' Administration be give additional authority in funds to carry out work they were already doing in heart disease, cancer and stroke.[36] It urged additional funds for Vocational Rehabilitations Administration and for the division of hospitals in the Bureau of Health Services;[37] it recommended increased authority for community and other outreach programs of the categorical disease institutes of NIH.[38] The Commission had special praise and urged substantial additional support for the National Library of Medicine:

The National Library of Medicine is the cornerstone of the National Library Network. Through its development of the world's largest collection of published medical literature and through its sponsorship and operation at the Medlars system, the largest computer-based information storage and retrieval system yet to be devised, the NLM has demonstrated its ability to improve the methodology and efficiency of this medical library network. But to exercise its proper leadership, the NLM required both broadened legislative authorities and additional funds for the purposes of strengthening and enlarging its intramural activities, and for the purpose of conducting the type of extramural support program the Commission has in mind."[39]

The Commission thought that some $30 million dollars in additional appropriations per year for five years would help the Library to move forward more strongly.

Thus, the commission had responded to the charge given to it by President Johnson: "...to recommend steps to reduce the incidence of these diseases through new knowledge and more complete utilization of the medical knowledge we already have."[40]

With its detailed, analysis, assessments and recommendations, the Commission delivered an exhortation matching the passion and conviction of the President to whom they reported:

> The Nation's strength derives from the strength of its people. A national investment in the prolonging of productive life for its people pays rich dividends in national productivity... Heart disease, cancer and stoke cut life short; they curtail the enjoyment of liberty; they make fearful the pursuit of happiness.[41]

> The President's Commission on Heart Disease, Cancer and Stroke bases its report on the conviction that the United States will measure up to greatness; that it will choose to continue and accelerate the forward thrust of medical research across new thresholds of discovery; and that it will resolve to make fully available the benefits of scientific knowledge to all those whose life and opportunity for individual fulfillment depend upon them.[42]

Notes:

1. U.S. Department of Health, Education of Welfare, "Health, Education and Welfare: Accomplishments, 1963-68, Problems and Challenges, and A Look to the Future," Report to President Lyndon B. Johnson, Dec. 1968, p.9.
2. Ibid.
3. President's Commission on Heart Disease, Cancer and Stroke, "Report to the President: A Program to Conquer Heart Disease, Cancer and Stroke," Vol. 1, Dec. 1964, (Appendix C) p.87.
4. Ibid.
5. Ibid.
6. Elizabeth Drew, "The Health Syndicate," Atlantic Monthly, Dec. 1967, p. 79.
7. Ibid.
8. Ibid.
9. Interview with Dr. DeBakey.
10. President's Commission on Heart Disease, Cancer and Stroke, "Report to the President," op. cit., p. 88.

11. Ibid., p. 89.

12. Ibid.,

13. See Elizabeth Drew, op.cit., and Stephen P. Strickland, Politics, Science and Dread Disease: A Short History of U.S. Biomedical Research Policy (Cambridge, Mass: Harvard University Press, 1972), esp. chapter III.

14. President's Commission on Heart Disease, Cancer and Stroke, "Report to the President, op. cit., appendix B, pp. 84-85.

15. Ibid., pp. 90-91

16. Ibid., p. 77. Elaboration included in President's Commission, "Report to the President," Vol. II, Feb. 1965.

17. President's Commission, "Report to the President," Vol I, op. cit., p. viii.

18. Ibid.

19. Ibid., p. xii.

20. Ibid., p. xiii.

21. Ibid., pp. 28-29

22. Ibid., p. 29

23. Ibid., pp. 29-30

24. Ibid., p. 30.

25. Ibid., p. 32.

26. Ibid., pp. 32-33.

27. Ibid., pp. 34-35.

28. Ibid.

29. Ibid.

30. Ibid., p. 35.

31. Ibid., pp. 35-36.

32. Ibid., pp. 36-37.

33. Ibid., p. 35.

34. Ibid., p. 64.

35. Ibid., pp. 31,40,41,43,44; p. 64.

36. Ibid., pp. 31-32, 50

37. Ibid., pp 64-65.

38. Ibid., p. xi.

39. Ibid., p. xiii.

40. Ibid.

Chapter 2

A Report Becomes A Bill, A Bill Becomes A Law

Public Law 89-239, The Heart Disease, Cancer and Stroke Amendments of 1965

While the Commission was taking its testimony and distilling its findings, the President was running for re-election. He was nominated by acclamation at the Democratic Convention in Atlantic City in August, 1964. With his ebullient running-mate, Senator Hubert Humphrey of Minnesota, barnstorming the country with equal fervor, Johnson was resoundingly reelected on November 4th. The landslide victory, and the expanded number of Democrats in the House and Senate which it helped to produce, insured that his legislative agenda would be met with approval. Indeed we have not seen anything like that agenda, nor the swiftness of favorable Congressional favorable disposition of it, since then.

The speed with which Lyndon Johnson built a case for doing what he wanted to do about the health of the nation, including heart disease, cancer and stroke, was to become a prime example of his legendary legislative prowess. In his health message to congress in February 1964, he had announced his intention to create a commission to "recommend steps to reduce the incidence of these diseases," and announced its first general meeting on April 17. In December the Commission delivered its report to the President. This permitted him, as he wished, to put its principal recommendations into a legislative proposal, to highlight the proposal in the course of his January 1965 State of the Union address, and to have the bill introduced in the first days of the first session of the 89th Congress.

The senior Senator from Alabama, Lister Hill, chairman of the Committee on Labor and Public Welfare, introduced the Bill, S. 596, in January 1965. Congressman Orrin Harris of Arkansas, Chairman of the House Inter-state and Foreign Commerce Committee introduced an identical bill, H.R. 3140, at the same time. Also introduced were companion measures for medical education, health facilities, libraries and other matters with which the Commission dealt.

The Congress -- or at least the Senate -- moved with impressive speed. Within a few weeks after the introduction of the bill, Senator Hill and his committee held hearings on February 9 and 10. Meanwhile, Hill had lined up witnesses representing the major traditional players; most of them supported the measure. In the course of formulating the legislation, the phrase "and other major diseases" had been added to the emphasis on heart disease, cancer and stroke. The American Cancer Society did not like the addition and asked for its deletion in the course of Senate consideration, apparently fearing a dilution of emphasis on the big three.[1]

The American Heart Association feared "the possibility of total domination by the medical schools."[2] The Association wanted to make sure that whatever form of governance regional medical centers and related complexes set up, such governing bodies would be truly representative of all major health care providers. The American Public Health Association expressed concern about the omission of the specific role of the state health departments.[3]

The Association of American Medical Colleges had multiple concerns. An early and continuing one dealt with health manpower. The initial reaction of some AAMC executive council members was that the emphasis on categorical diseases and developing more physicians to deal with them would both strain the aggregate physician capacity of the country and skew it in the direction of these categories. Dr. Douglas Bond, Dean of the Western Reserve University School of Medicine in Cleveland, said: "A more rigid structure than we now have would be of questionable value since the major medical centers are already concentrated in the three diseases covered in the report... our care and clinical research are already focused there."[4] From an executive session of the Executive Council of the AAMC on February 5, 1965: "It was the consensus of the Executive Council that S.596 is premature as it will cause a further drain on the increasing shortage of physicians (manpower)."[5]

The AAMC strongly preferred to see Congress first pass a bill to help overcome the health manpower shortage, and then take up the matter of extending the knowledge and skills of physicians attached to sophisticated medical centers out to community hospitals. However, being realistic as well as principled, the Executive Council in short order adopted the following position: "Since it appears that S. 596 will be passed, emphasis must be place on the importance of S. 595 (Health Manpower Bill) going hand in hand with it and also in raising the proposed amounts of funds to be allocated for educating medical students.... The Executive Council [proposes] that the AAMC's general position stress the importance of the role of the university, the medical center and the medical school in overall decisions as well as operation of the proposed complex."[6] (Apparently, Executive Committee leaders and staff had not had time to read the DeBakey Commission report.)

The next day, February 6, Dr. William Stewart, Assistant to the Special Assistant (Health) to the Secretary of the Department of Health Education and Welfare -- very shortly to become Surgeon General of the Public Health Service -- came to the AAMC meeting to talk about the President's message, "Advancing the Nation's Health". Because Senator Hill was in fact going to hold hearings on the heart disease, cancer and stroke amendments of 1965 within days, the discussion was focused on that legislation. Stewart assuaged the concern of the medical school administrators by addressing head on the matter of "the increasing shortage of physicians in the United States, especially of those knowledgeable in the newer developments... service and training institutions must be linked together in order to employ as efficiently as possible the manpower available."[7] But he pushed a little bit as well: Because the best medical centers, usually attached to excellent medical schools, set the standard for quality of patient care, the medical centers therefore must be "the vehicle by which the quality of care is upgraded" [by] "getting the latest facilities and techniques into communities."[8]

The AAMC seemed to be impressed by Dr. Stewart's logic and presentation. They were very possibly reassured by his indication that the program would move cautiously. For example, the bill called for an appropriation of $50 million in 1966 and the Department's goal, within a year of enactment, was only four complexes.[9] Continuing in its cooperative mode, the AAMC decided to organize regional meetings of medical schools leaders for discussion of the several bills, and what they would mean separately and together.

Not all physicians representing important constituencies agreed with the assessments of the DeBakey Commission, the President, and physicians representing the Department of Health Education and Welfare on why the legislation was needed. Dr. George E. Burkett, Jr., Chairman of the Board of the American Academy of General Practice and President of the Kansas Medical Society stated: "I do not see how the system proposed in the report will directly benefit the general practitioner, who already has knowledge of the practical advances, and is increasingly active in post-graduate training... The so called lag is not a problem, the practicing physician is fully capable of keeping up with significant advances if he wants to."[10]   Dr. Joseph Garland, Editor of The New England Journal of Medicine, asserted: "I do not look for immediate practical value from programs such as this. The slow process of assimilation and sifting must take place in the application of any medical advances."[11]

Dean Bond of Western Reserve fretted about the practicality of a disease-oriented plan of attack. "It tends to alienate people working on different diseases. And we already have too much of this non-communication. Making a distinction between heart disease and stroke, for instance, encourages the very fragmentation we are trying to overcome."[12] To which Dr. DeBakey replied: "Patients don't die from a general medical condition; they die from a disease." He continued: "Diseases occur in categories, we classify them, and it is logical to have a program concentrating on the three most devastating diseases."[13] Besides, while the Commission thought stroke deserved independent emphasis, its report had stated up front its connection to "the heart itself and blood vessels serving the body, its place in the spectrum of cardiovascular-renal diseases."[14]

The Senate committee worked through or around some of these critiques. In June, the bill was reported out of Committee and sent to the Senate for consideration. The bill recommended all basic elements of the original proposal and provided authorization of $650 million for the next four years.

Meanwhile, a bigger controversy had been brewing, one about which Dr. DeBakey and his commission colleagues should have had some clue. Dr. Hugh Hussey, representative of the American Medical Association on the Commission, resigned in September 1964, just as the Commission's work was being completed. Shortly after the Commission reported to the President, and before the Congress commenced its hearings on the legislation, the AMA released a staff report which contained a bombshell: "The President's Commission on Heart, Cancer and Stroke -- and by inference the bills being considered in the Congress of the United States -- actually propose to reorganize medical services... The degree of implicit federalization and coercion are novel."[15] And, for the AMA, completely unacceptable.

The AMA, like some other critics, disagreed that there was a serious lag between new medical concepts and diagnostic and treatment modes and their widespread application by practicing physicians. And it did not like the idea of designated centers or complexes. Dr. Irving Page, Editor of Modern Medicine detailed the controversies in the June 1965 issue of this magazine. While laying out some pro's and cons, and the opinions of the opposing experts as to the merits and demerits of the proposal, his reservations were more than clear: "As a taxpayer I do not want to subsidize a large portion of the medical facilities in this country... The Senate hearings have been superficial, without regard for the long-range effects the commission report might have if enacted into law."[16] The bill was ambiguous and Dr. Page did not consider the AAMC`s positions to be principled: "A number of medical schools have taken to the drawing boards and taken to 'chameleon plans,' which would both attract large federal funds and still avoid federal support of medical practice."[17] "It is time for wisdom and restraint. The urge to get the money now and think later has nothing to recommend it." All professional groups should debate the matter, and the "firm result of these debates should then be made available to Congress and to the people."[18]

In the Bulletin of the Los Angeles County Medical Association, Dr. Ian McDonald called the DeBakey Commission Report "the real blueprint for the federal take-over of medical research, teaching and practice."[19]

If the private practice of medicine becomes virtually extinct in this decade, the name of one individual will be recognized as the chief architect of its obliteration. No politician or legislator, no King or Anderson, no planner of the welfare state will have this distinction. Even the would-be Creator of the "Great Society" will not be given primary credit. The elimination of the independent practicing physician, of partnerships and group practice in the United States, of any form of medical service not subservient to the Federal Government, will have been the achievement of one of our own profession--a specialist in cardiovascular surgery in a Texas university hospital, one Michael DeBakey.[20]

By the time Dr. McDonald's pronouncement appeared in print, in November 1965, the Commission report had been substantially transformed and a program of regional cooperative arrangements had been adopted by Congress. But the Los Angeles physicians were still wary. Even though they admitted that the final law was "only a shadow version of the DeBakey Report," they cautioned: "There's no guarantee that the more ominous portions of the report will not become law in future years in view of the welfaristic trend of events in Washington and Sacramento."[21]

The President of the AMA, Dr. Charles L. Hudson subsequently commented:

We have inferred that this, a closed entity of indeterminate size, excluding others already practicing in the area, was intended to demonstrate in a disparaging way perhaps the inadequacies of our physicians. Believing the premises upon which these actions were based to be false, and concerned that this was a revolutionary change in the system of health care not in the public interest, the AMA did not support the legislation.[22]

The latter may be considered as one of the great understatements in the contentious politics of national health policy from the 1950's into the 1990's. Many of those involved in the Regional Medical Programs idea and proposed legislation, and in broader health policy circles, reported that when the AMA leadership finally focused on the DeBakey Commission report and resulting legislation, they "went ballistic."

Simultaneously, the American Academy of General Practice launched its assault. It called the proposed program "an unparalleled threat to the private practice of medicine, a threat that is of far greater magnitude than any associated with Social Security health plans."[23]

The AMA took its case directly to the White House. The Association had spent much of its time since the President's re-election fighting Medicare and Medicaid. It apparently had not paid much attention to the heart, cancer and stroke legislation. Regarding Medicare and Medicaid, AMA cooperation was still needed to insure its appropriate implementation, and its leaders were, like those of all other professional associations, consulted about the larger proposals. The AMA's position was that it would not cooperate in the implementation of Medicare and Medicaid unless the Senate bill proposing regional heart, cancer and stroke medical programs was dramatically changed: "We reported to President Johnson our belief that passing this, the Senate version, upon the heels of Medicare would be repugnant to the physicians of the country and would adversely affect their attitude toward any and all federal support programs, especially Medicare."[24]

The most important change made in the course of the negotiations with the AMA, and its allies in other organizations and in the Congress, was this: Rather than calling for the identification of existing and future medical complexes with specialized capacities "centers of excellence," it instead envisioned a network of "cooperative arrangements" voluntarily entered into by a range of health care providers. Whether or not this change in language and emphasis, hence in concept, made the critical difference in the development and ultimate demise of Regional Medical Programs cannot be known. Why the designation of such centers was so threatening to the AMA, viewed from a quarter of a century later, is still mildly puzzling. Dr. Hudson makes the opposition sound too philosophical: "Inherent in this recognition is the hazard that judgments of high position in a vertical scale will disparage any other contributor to the whole scheme."[25]

Dr. DeBakey remarked that he spent much time traveling around to medical meetings to try to correct doctors' "misunderstanding" of the purposes of the legislation and of the DeBakey Commission. One of those who seemed to listen was Congressman Tim Lee Carter of Kentucky, the ranking Republican member of the House State and Foreign Commerce Committee and earlier a practicing physician. With assurances from Dr. DeBakey and others, including spokesmen from the Administration, Congressman Carter said that he would join in supporting a revised bill in the House.

The AMA proposed most of the twelve amendments added to the House bill before Congressman Harris got the agreement of his committee colleagues to bring the legislation to the floor. The most important changes in the House bill were these: "regional medical complexes" and "coordinated arrangements" became "regional medical programs" and "cooperative arrangements."[26] And there was one other critically important addition to the language: "To accomplish these ends without interfering with the patterns, or the methods of financing, of patient care or professional practice."[27]

The bill finally enacted in law, in October, 1965, Public Law 89-239, adhered to the House Committee's language. It authorized appropriations of $50 million for the first fiscal year (ending June 30, 1966), $90 million for the second, and $200 million for the third (ending June 30, 1968) -- a total of $340 million in contrast to the Senate bill's $650 million.[28] The amounts actually appropriated didn't even approach the authorized ceilings.

The indefatigable, experienced and politically sophisticated Wilbur Cohen, the HEW Under Secretary who had helped President Roosevelt pass Social Security in 1935 and helped Lyndon Johnson pass a plethora of health bills in the 89th Congress, later said that the opposition of the AMA and the American Academy of General Practice to the Senate bill was such that "to come up with acceptable language for the House bill taxed all the ingenuity I gained from thirty years of legislative experience."[29]

Dr. Philip R. Lee, who joined as Assistant Secretary for Health in mid-1965, remembers Cohen pacing back and forth in his stocking feet late into the summer evenings that year, trying out new language on any staff members still in the office.[30]

Cohen's own philosophy of doing something practical for people, as well as working to overcome political problems to achieve a successful legislative outcome, were evident in all his remarks, before, during and after the enactment of the Heart, Cancer and Stroke Amendments of 1965. Periodically he invoked the conceptual approach of his boss, HEW Secretary John W. Gardner on the subject of "creative federalism." He quoted Gardner's reassuring words: "We have a multiplicity of institutions, public and private (universities, hospitals, etc.) and we have no intention of submerging their identity in some rigorous master plan. The solution is to be found in new forms of cooperation among the institutions."[31]

But even after working out critical legislative compromises, the Undersecretary thought the fundamental difference between those trying to help LBJ form a Great Society and the vigorous and relentless opponents of it, including the American Medical Association, should not be obscured:

> Some have argued that there is an inconsistency or even conflict between high quality and wide-spread use. They believe that excellence is such a rare and tender flower that it can only bloom in special and carefully protected environments. They have suggested that we can lose everything by trying to reproduce what requires the most skilled craftsmanship. This point of view, I believe, is contrary to our national history and commitment. I think we have the capabilities as a society to make the very best available to all our people. This is our national goal.[32]

Notes:

1. "Evolution or Revolution in American Medicine," Modern Medicine, (Special Report), June 21, 1965, p. 14.
2. Ibid.
3. Ibid.
4. Ibid., pp. 20,23.
5. Association of American Medical Colleges, Executive Council Meeting Minutes, (Executive Session), February 5, 1965, p.7.
6. Ibid., p. 8.
7. "AAMC Proceedings for 1965," Journal of Medical Education, Vol. 41, June 1966, p. 527.
8. AAMC, Executive Council Meeting Minutes (Open Session), Feb. 5, 1965, p. 5.
9. Ibid.
10. "Evolutions or Revolution in American Medicine," op. cit., pp. 26, 24.
11. Ibid., p. 29.
12. Ibid.
13. Ibid.
14. The President's Commission on Heart Disease, Cancer and Stroke, "Report to the President," Vol. I, Dec. 1964, p. 84.
15. "Evolution and Revolution in American Medicine," op. cit., p.16.
16. Ibid., p. 91.
17. Ibid.
18. Ibid., pp. 91-92.
19. Bulletin of the Los Angeles County Medical Association, Nov. 1965.
20. Ibid.
21. Ibid
22. Ibid.
23. Modern Medicine, June 1965, op. cit. p.16.
24. "Proceedings," op. cit. p. 7.

22

25. Ibid.

26. Public Law 89-239, 89th Congress, 3.596. Oct. 6. 1965.

27. Ibid.

28. Ibid.

29. U.S.D.H.E.W., "Proceedings: Conference on Regional Medical Programs, Jan. 1967,11 p. 10.

30. Interview with Dr. Phillip R. Lee, Aug. 31, 1993, Cosmos Club.

31. U.S.D.H.E.W., "Proceedings," op. cit. p.10.

32. Ibid.

Chapter 3

Organization

In 1965 alone, twelve health laws were enacted by the 89th Congress and signed by the President. He and his Department of Health Education and Welfare had initiated most of them. Each required an organizational base. Many such were long-standing, because some of the laws, including extensions to the Hill-Burton Act, were amendments to programs that had been administered for years by the same office, division, branch or bureau.

Medicare and Medicaid were the biggest challenges. Medicare would naturally go to the Social Security Administration; it was designed that way and based on that system. The worrying thing about Medicaid was that although it was to be a cooperative program between the federal government and the states, it would be large -- though not nearly so large as the President had indicated and the states had expected. Where to lodge it was a challenge to the HEW directorate. One of their concerns was that none of the traditional bureaus of the Public Health Service had any direct experience, at least since the 1930's, in dealing with poor people.[1]

Regarding Regional Medical Programs, created by the Heart Disease, Cancer and Stroke Amendments of 1965, there was on-going discussion. Before the proposed legislation had left the Senate Committee, Senator Hill had added language specifying that RMP be located in the National Institutes of Health. Between that point and the final passage of the Bill in October, that specification had been deleted. Many discussions were held; there were pros and cons about where to put it. NIH was of course one possibility, but this depended in significant part on whether its director, Dr. James Shannon, wanted the program housed in his agency.

As a general proposition, Dr. Shannon resisted any extension of the central role of NIH, the support or conduct of biomedical research. The only exception he made was where developmental aspects of such research were to be carried out in medical schools and graduate departments of universities or related laboratories, which, with their faculties, were the principal and preeminent partners in the aggregate national biomedical research enterprise.[2]

The new program, by statute, was required to involve medical schools centrally. Both from Dr. Shannon's point of view and that of others involved in making final decisions, NIH was virtually the only federal agency which had real experience in dealing with medical schools.[3] On the other hand, the medical schools were required to establish linkages with communities in their areas and such linkages were few and far between. Physicians, medical school deans, and policy makers alike knew this to be true. Some said it was outside the experience of medical schools to have such links. Dean Stanley Olson of Baylor said of that university's medical center: "It was almost as though here was an island of excellence and everything out there was 'other'. It was something that we had no direct contact with. Sure, physicians would refer patients and we would send the patients back with information about what had been seen and done." But with most communities, "we really didn't have any linkage."[4]

Despite Dr. Shannon's reluctance to get involved in anything remotely approaching the delivery of services, he thought there were two fundamental questions that should govern the answer of where RMP should be housed within the Department: First, what agency could swiftly incorporate and effectively carry out the mandate of overseeing the development of Regional Medical Programs? The Bureau of State Services did not have extensive and consistent relations with medical schools. Second, if NIH did not take charge, would a new, burgeoning program under some other aegis cause a problem for NIH and its constituency? The NIH was, in that period, the most vibrant, dynamic health agency in the government. In the end Dr. Shannon decided that if there was to be a significant, and possibly very large, new federal health-related program -- related to the fruits of medical research -- perhaps it would be better to have it under his control than outside it.[5]

While Dr. Shannon pondered the matter, the Surgeon General, Dr.

Luther L. Terry, formed a committee of senior agency and bureau officials to consider it. When decision time came, the designated NIH representative, acquainted with his director's ambivalence but not with his final decision, voted against putting RMP in NIH. His vote tilted the balance in the wrong direction. Dr. Shannon called Dr. Terry and somehow the vote was reversed. RMP would go to NIH.[6]

Dr. Robert Q. Marston, Dean of the Medical School of the University of Mississippi, had from time to time talked with friends and acquaintances in the federal establishment about taking a federal position. He had been strenuously engaged in building up his medical school and had turned down other opportunities. But the possibility of creating a program, centered in part in medical schools but reaching across the country to enhance the capacity to deliver first-rate care to people, was appealing. Further, as if to presage larger possibilities in the future as well as to emphasize the importance of the program to the host agency, Dr. Shannon suggested that if Dr. Marston were to accept the challenge, he would be designated Associate Director of the National Institutes of Health as well as Director of the Office of Regional Medical Programs. Marston decided to accept and came to Washington in early 1966.[7]

The Public Health Service, from its earliest days and certainly from the New Deal through the Great Society, was populated with extraordinarily talented physicians and other health professionals. It was out of the PHS bureaus that some of the most distinguished directors of NIH institutes and programs had emerged. This was especially true after World War II and in the 1950's, as NIH -- a PHS bureau -- entered its glorious decade of expanding missions, vastly expanding appropriations, and rapidly increased need for experienced people. So it was natural and valuable that virtually every member of the principal staff of the Division of Regional Medical Programs of NIH had already been in NIH or some other part of the Public Health Service.

One of the principal conceptualizers of the program as it got underway was Karl Yordy, a young man on the staff of Dr. Shannon. Among other advantages of his central involvement were his earlier service in the old Bureau of the Budget and his training, at Harvard University, in public administration. If ever a new federal program would tax the practical administrative capacity of those in charge and require an understanding of the constitutional structure of governmental arrangements generally, RMP would do so. Yordy filled both bills. How do you administer from the top a voluntary cooperative system which is supposed to be energized from the bottom up? Others were recruited from other parts of the PHS and government -- Dr. Margaret Sloan, Charles Elsenroth, Ed Friedlander, Mark Phillips, Steven Akerman, Dan Zwick. An important person from the field was brought in, Dr. William D. Mayer, then at the University of Missouri School of Medicine, who became, early in 1966, the first Associate Director of RMP for Continuing Education.[8]

The first task Dr. Marston had was in completing the National Advisory Council of RMP, mandated by law. Nominees came from a variety of sources, and Dr. Shannon and Dr. Stewart were very much involved in the selection. Indeed, Dr. Stewart by law served as Chair of the Council. Its members were impressive individually as well as in the aggregate. They included Dr.Leonidas Berry, a practicing physician and clinical professor who also served as the elected President of the National Medical Association, the Black physicians' counterpart to the AMA; Mary Bunting, President of Radcliffe College (the only woman on the Advisory Council); Charles Hitch, Vice President for Administration of the University of California; John Hogness, Dean of the School of Medicine of the University of Washington (later to be that university's president, President of the Association of American Medical Colleges and first President of the Institute of Medicine); Dr. William J. Peeples, Health Commissioner for the State of Maryland and his counterpart Dr. Mack John Holtz of Virginia. The connective tissue of institutional memory, if there was need of such, were present in the persons of Dr. Mike DeBakey and Dr. J. Willis Hurst.[9] Within six months the staff and council had established guidelines for the program; created outreach and interactive communications groups to give advice to regions and potential regions; defined such regions principally by letting regions define themselves; confirmed a grants submission, review, and decision making process; and not only announced the availability of planning grants but actually made some.

Indeed, the National Advisory Council awarded seven such grants in April 1966, three more in June, eight more in August, and in November approved sixteen additional applications. Within a year not only was the government organized, but 34 Regional Medical Programs were in business. It was estimated that "the total population covered by planning activities represented 90% of the nation."[10] One additional big challenge, was that, even as the directorate continued to define and delineate, explain and encourage the fledgling enterprise, the same group was also aggregating and then summarizing information on how the program was doing. For the law required that an evaluation of the program be made and submitted to the President and the Congress by the Surgeon General within two years.

Surely this time pressure had positive benefits for the rapid development of Regional Medical Programs despite placing enormous pressure on the staff. Dr. Marston and Dr. Stewart followed President Johnson's example, appointing a special ad hoc subcommittee of the advisory council in the fall of 1966, to develop a report to be presented, in six to nine months.[11] To do so, a national conference of some 650 persons, representing a broad spectrum of health and related groups throughout the nation, was held in January 1967 to discuss and exchange views on the development of the program.[12]

In June of 1967, Surgeon General Stewart submitted such a report with recommendations for continuation of the program but with some changes.

Dr. Stewart's report was straightforward in its restatement of fundamental purposes, acknowledgment of the restrictions held sacrosanct by organized medicine, and emphasis of the pioneering nature of the program. For example:

Regional Medical Programs put into practice [the rule] that essential responsibility and power for the improvement of health services should be exercised locally...with freedom and flexibility to do those things necessary to achieve goals of each program provided...[However] the law does not allow support of isolated projects, however meritorious if they do not contribute to new or improved regional cooperative arrangements.[13]

Or again:

New systems are being sought amid diverse geographic and social circumstances that will make available to all the people medical services for heart disease, cancer and stroke and related diseases that are excellent in quality and adequate in quantity, while preserving the diversity and largely private character of our medical care process.[14]

It surely did not occasion surprise in any quarter that the Surgeon General of the U.S. Public Health Service, backed by the National Institutes of Health, the Regional Medical Programs already established, and most of the 650 participants consulated in the course of preparing his report, recommended that Public Law 89-239 be extended. The Surgeon General would have preferred a five-year extension, and hoped the President and Congress would grant it, so that "the long-term commitment of the kind and quality of people and the full participation of all affected institutions, which are essential to the program's success, be insured."[15] That concern -- whether the federal government would, once more, start something and then back away from its commitment -- persists even today, despite the fact that government programs at any level, but particularly at the national level, are rarely cut off. That the 103rd Congress in 1993 terminated funding for the Super-Collider is one of the rarer instances of this phenomenon in our national history.

Yet the Surgeon General was obviously reflecting the reality with which he and the Division of Regional Medical Programs were dealing when he stated: "Individuals undertaking regional planning have reported that uncertainty about the program's future is a serious obstacle in recruiting well-qualified persons..." and that "some institutions and agencies have been reluctant to embark upon a course of action, whatever it's promise and potential, without reasonable assurance the program would be continued."[16]

The specific modifications recommended -- reversing the ban on paying for facilities construction, specifying authority for the support of inter-regional activities, the inclusion of dentists including their referral of patients to Regional Medical Programs, and permission for intergovernmental activities (e.g., Veteran's Administration) -- were all natural, even if, in some instances, these were of more concern to particular constituencies than stemming from the overall experience of the first two years.

The identification of some problems that marked the early experience of RMP was not unusual. For example, Dr. Stewart reported that: "Some medical leaders seriously questioned whether the university is an appropriate focus for the leadership of these cooperative efforts."[17] The doubts included whether RMP responsibilities might divert medical school resources from teaching and research functions; whether "medical school leadership will result in domination or absorption of other health resources by the medical school"; and "about the capacity of university medical centers to expand their administrative frameworks to encompass a Regional Medical Program."[18]

There were other problems not identified in the report. Only a year earlier on June 27, 1966 President Johnson had invited Dr. Shannon and directors of all the institutes of the National Institutes of Health to the White House for a general discussion. Without indicating in advance any particular agenda, the President stunned the medical research leaders and their constituencies, the universities and medical schools, by asking whether "too much energy was being spent on basic research and not enough on translating laboratory findings into tangible benefits for the American people."[19] The President asked the NIH directorate to consider this question and, if necessary, to reshape their priorities in order to get maximum results.

As a journalist observer wrote: "The President's initiative... caused an explosion among the scientists and universities. They took it to mean that the Lasker forces were in the saddle, that support for categorical research and development would be substituted for basic research by an anti-intellectual, unsophisticated president who could never understand such a thing."[20]

Two months later, Secretary of Health Education and Welfare John Gardner invited all NIH advisors and consultants, including persons involved in Regional Medical Programs, to come to a meeting at the Department. He assured them that there was not a fixed federal health dollar for which basic research and applied and developmental activities and delivery of services had to compete. Instead, he suggested, the government was probably going to spend an increasing amount of its revenues on health. One of the things Gardner emphasized was that the administration's dedication to such new programs as the heart, cancer and stroke centers and Regional Medical Programs would mean that "the future of one or another form of university extension activity in the medical field is going to be very lively indeed."[21] Implicitly, the suggestion was that through all such programs, the university was not only to be counted on as a critically important partner but as the recipient of continued federal funds in a variety of forms. A year later the President helicoptered out to the Bethesda campus of NIH to thank Dr. Shannon for his report claiming that 60% of NIH monies already went for applied research and specifying items of medical progress in the last two decades. The President praised the NIH directorate, staff and grantees, and called the enterprise "a billion dollar success story."[22]

It turned out to be true that NIH appropriations kept increasing annually, as did the aggregate federal dollars going to medical schools and universities. It is also a fact that when Regional Medical Programs were reauthorized in 1967 as requested by the Surgeon General, the authorized appropriation ceilings included in them posed a new hazard. For the specified amounts gradually but obviously came to be at odds with fiscal realities. Would RMP really become a $300 billion investment?

Notes:

1. Interview with Dr. Phillip R. Lee.
2. Interview with Karl Yordy, August 26, 1993.
3. Ibid.
4. Interview with Dr. Olson, Collection of National Library of Medicine.
5. Interview with Karl Yordy.
6. Ibid.
7. Oral History Interview with Dr. Marston, conducted by Stephen Goodell, for Lyndon B. Johnson Library, Austin Texas, April 18, 1969.
8. U. S. Department of Health, Education and Welfare, "Proceedings: Conference on Regional Medical Programs, Jan. 967," p. 95.
9. ibid., p. 94.
10. Ibid., p. 12.
11. U.S. Department of Health, Education and Welfare, "Report of Regional Medical Programs to the President and the Congress," submitted by William H. Stewart, M.D., June 1967, p. 61.
12. U.S.D.H.E.W., "Proceedings: Conference on Regional Medical Programs, op. cit.
13. U.S.D.H.E.W., "Report on Regional Medical Programs," June 1967, pp. 7-8.
14. Ibid., p. 8.
15. Ibid., p. 32.
16. Ibid.
17. Ibid., p. 29.
18. Ibid.
19. Stephen P. Strickland, Politics, Science and Dread Disease, (Cambridge, Mass: Harvard University Press, 1972), p. 207.
20. Elizabeth Drew, "The Health Syndicate," Atlantic Monthly, Dec. 1967, p. 81.

21. Strickland, op. cit., pp. 208-209.
22. Ibid., p. 209.

Chapter 4

Regions: Delineations and Definitions

When we begin to look for the perfect definition of a region either as a principle of organizing medical services or principle of organizing any services, we soon realize the tremendous complexity of American life.[1]

The regional approach to health care is relatively new in American social history and not very old anywhere in the western world. The British, in 1920, considered a proposal by the Minister of Health -- the Dawson Report -- to construct a network of primary and secondary hospitals linked to teaching hospitals as the most effective way both of integrating hospital services and equalizing the quality of them throughout the country. The plan was gradually effectuated in the decades following, and the British model has since served as an example for regionalization attempts in other countries.[2]

In the United States, the Committee on the Costs of Medical Care, established in 1927, worked on a comprehensive conceptual plan for the delivery of enhanced health care in American which contained, among other provisions, major elements of a regionalized program of health services. Presented in 1932, the plan called for non-profit community medical centers, in cities with populations of 15,000 or more, linked to and served by physicians in (presumably for-profit) group medical practice.[3]

Meanwhile, in 1931, the Bingham Associates Fund, working with Tufts Medical School and the Pratt Diagnostic Hospital in Boston, supported a new regional system of health services throughout Maine and part of Massachusetts. The plan permitted local physicians, who were uncertain about particular diagnostic problems and complex surgical possibilities to refer patients   directly to Tufts or Pratt for more sophisticated care. The system included regular consultations between practicing physicians in smaller communities and teaching physicians and clinicians at Tufts and Pratt in radiology and electrocardiography as well as in diagnosis. Graduating physicians were sent for internships in community hospitals in Lewiston and Bangor, Maine, armed with fresh information about particular diseases and other medical problems and how to deal with them. In short, "the Medical School thus entered into direct support of individual practitioners, with the aim of improving the quality of medical practice."[4] The Tufts New England program continued for 35 years, being expanded, modified, and otherwise dynamic in its dimensions and its emphases during that period, until it became a program incorporated under the aegis of regional medical programs. And yet, at least one astute and comprehensive observer of medical care and health policy, Dr. William Kissick, has commented that, at least in the early days, the Tufts/New England program met with only limited success.[5]

The University of Iowa Hospitals and Clinics located in Iowa City became the first Regional Medical Program prototype west of the Mississippi River. With its affiliated schools of medicine and nursing, the institution historically has trained most of the physicians, nurses and other health professionals in the state. And from the 1920's when its ambulance service started, it has been the logistical and technological link among the principal hospitals and physicians throughout Iowa.[6]

Other regional approaches in health and hospital care involved large metropolitan areas. These included the Hospital Review and Planning Council of Southern New York, created in 1938; the Rochester, N.Y. Hospital Council, incorporated in 1939; and the Columbus, Ohio Federation, incorporated in 1945.

The Council of Rochester Regional Hospitals was, as in the case of the New England/Tufts arrangement, supported by a private sector foundation, the Commonwealth Fund. Its purposes were: "Continuing education for all categories of health personnel, advisory service in clinical medicine and hospital administration, joint hospital services on a regional basis, and standards for hospital operation." At its center was Rochester University Hospital.[7]

For the country as a whole, the intrepid leaders of the US Public Health Service in the 1940s were also thinking in regional terms. The PHS Medical Director, Dr. Joseph Mountain, working with and encouraged by Dr. Thomas Parran, the Surgeon General, recommended that regional health service areas be created across the country to address the problem of the "lack of uniformity" of general hospitals throughout the nation.[8] But it was not only lack of uniformity that troubled those looking at the provision of medical care in general hospitals. A more challenging phenomenon was that the frontiers of medicine and biology had been greatly extended during the war years. The most dramatic example of a medical treatment advance was penicillin, first used widely and effectively on the battlefield and in military hospitals, and now capable of being mass-produced. Surgery had also achieved new and exquisite standards.

Inspired by such medical breakthroughs and encouraged by Mary Lasker and Florence Mahoney, Senator Claude Pepper of Florida in 1944 held hearings on the future of medicine and biomedical research. These became a landmark in governmental and public discussion of the role of the Federal Government in supporting biomedical science research, and scientific research generally, and of how to extend the benefits of some of the major advances to the broader populace.[9] It was in this context that Dr. Mountain and his colleagues "attempted to project a plan for an integrated scheme of hospitals and related facilities to cover every section of the nation."[10] Through this system, they believed, one of the principal impediments to providing good medical care could be overcome:

Lack of hospital construction has the effect of depriving many physicians of opportunities for continuing education afforded by professional associations in well-conducted clinics and staff meetings. For the same reason, they may be denied the use of equipment other than what they can afford to purchase individually. Rural practitioners, especially, have been isolated from advances in modern medical science and technology. Rather than become victims of this situation, physicians and other medical personnel concentrate in centers of wealth and population, thus increasing the maldistribution of medical service.[11]

The Mountain Report, endorsed by the Surgeon General and presented to the Congress as well as to the President, became one of the building blocks for the Hill-Burton Hospital Survey and Construction Act of 1946. This act, in turn, was the reference point for many subsequent federal health programs. Its principal features were: specification of national goals and standards; grants to states for these purposes, with funds going to community and sometimes private hospitals; shared funding, with states having to match the federal investment; and the requirement for surveys of need and patterns of care before particular projects were funded.

Those conceptualizing and subsequently implementing the regional medical programs in the mid-1960s used Hill-Burton as one important antecedent. But as such it had serious limitations. Like Hill-Burton, the RMP legislation posited a clear national goal, but the new the program was supposed to serve populations in particular areas notwithstanding political boundaries, including state boundaries.

In the new program, grants were not to be made to states. Public Law 89-239 required: "1) each region should be large enough to include (or warrant the inclusion of) such an amount and variety of resources for health services that, when they are properly integrated, the region will be self-sufficient for most purposes; 2) each region should be small enough to make the administrative center or any other unique feature accessible to all parts of the region. Regional populations might vary from one-half to ten million, and distribution from center to periphery might vary from 20-25 to 250 or more miles."[12] The question was whether the emphasis on the functional purposes would run up against the problem of geographic boundaries.

It is no wonder that in the first guidelines offered to those attempting to form regional medical programs, the guideline drafters suggested that regional medical program groups should define their own regions. Indeed, most of them did, taking into account both practical, nonpolitical jurisdictional matters such as where people ordinarily went to get medical care or where the physicians referred them, which was often across state lines; and, on the other hand, geographical and other political delineations.

It was obviously the view of the policy makers that in typical, optimistic, largely wonderful American fashion, regional medical programs would be developed pragmatically. So the first task of the early organizers of particular regional medical programs, including their advisory councils, was to deal with the challenge of constructing regional medical programs in the correct demographic, geographic, functional and political proportions. As Paul Ilvisaker observed, delineating a region "is to add a territorial ambition to an otherwise complicated existence." And all who had ever attempted such delineations felt a nagging truth in the further observation that a region is "that area which is safely larger or smaller than the last one whose problems we couldn't solve."[13]

Fortunately, in some instances the delineation of region was simple. Usually, the easy cases were the ones in which state boundaries encompassed a few strong institutions which acted as centrifugal magnets within the state. These included states with a single medical school, graduates of which stayed to practice within the state and whose affiliated university hospital was the center of excellence. Thus Alabama, Iowa, Kansas, Arizona, and a handful of others would turn out to have a relatively easy time of it.

This pattern was not universally true. For example, Connecticut, with one old, distinguished, private medical school, Yale, and one regional state institution, the University of Connecticut Medical School, had difficulties from the beginning. Yale had never been Connecticut-centered even though it was Connecticut-based. Yet when regional medical programs held out the promise of the creation of a state-encompassing network of health and medical activity, the old school did not want to simply yield the state to the new school simply because it, Yale, was "a national institution."

Other difficult delineations occurred in the wide open spaces of the country. The requirement of medical schools being centrally involved in regional programs produced frustration in Nevada and Idaho. "What are we supposed to do?," Dr. Lee Castle Hilman asked of the Office of Regional Medical Programs in 1967. "We don't have a medical school."[14]

The biggest dilemma and challenge lay in large metropolitan areas not contained completely within state boundaries. Everybody knew that lots of people in Northeast Mississippi and Southeast Arkansas went to doctors or hospitals in Memphis and that people in Southwestern Illinois went to St. Louis. Then there were New York and Philadelphia. They both had a number of medical schools located within their jurisdictions; each of these had affiliated teaching hospitals which often treated some portions of populations for one problem while others treated the same patient for different ones. The planners and policy makers, and those really focused on the regional patterns of health care delivery and education, hoped things would work out in a natural way. In most cases they did.

Then there were the implications of other federal programs and efforts that had to be contended with. For example, a few months after RMP was authorized, Congress passed the Comprehensive of Health Planning Act of 1966 which charged states with planning the future of health resources in their overall jurisdiction and subregions within them.[15] This legislation had been seen by some as giving a nod both to state health agencies and to the traditional U.S. Public Health Service arrangements, for most PHS programs dealt with state authority.

Ironically, in other programs of the Kennedy and Johnson years, it was the conservatism in state governments in a variety of fields that had prompted the government to devise programs for the delivery of funds directly to communities. This included prominently programs of the War on Poverty, many run by the Office of Economic Opportunity. In some of these programs there was not just an anti-state government tendency, but an anti-government tendency: community groups with no structural connection to even local governments were often the preferred recipients of federal largesse.

Lyndon Johnson's assistants occasionally explained what seemed to be competing purposes and activities of various of his policies or programs — said to have common goals but forced to compete with each other for resources -- as a matter of consciously produced or induced "creative tension."[16] In any case, some Great Society programs favored state structures, some favored municipal governments, some favored community groups, and some favored entities organized along functional lines. Regional Medical Programs, with their fundamental functional purpose, had to deal with all these contending factors.

Cooperative Arrangements

Still another definition challenged the imagination and the pragmatism of regional medical programs and their advisory councils.

This was the requirement and the objective, specified in the language of the law, regarding "the establishment of regional cooperative arrangements among medical schools, research institutions and hospitals for research and training (including continuing education) and for related demonstrations of patient care..."[17] Other sections of the law (and the committee reports which comprise the legislative history) added that "all organizations and groups concerned with realizing the purposes of the law should be involved including 'medical societies, health departments, voluntary agencies, other health professions and individuals concerned with health.'" Members of regional advisory groups must be "broadly representative."[18]

This challenge contained within it one of the most potent elements of the new law and new program. Since no one knew precisely what was involved in a cooperative arrangement, beyond the illustrative indication of the kinds of institutions and professional types that ought to be involved, the only thing for representatives of such groups and institutions to do was to sit down together and talk about the development of cooperative arrangements. There was no question as to the purpose of such cooperative arrangements. It was "to afford medical profession and medical institutions of the nation... the opportunity of making available to their patients to latest treatment in heart disease, cancer, stroke and related diseases."[19]

Dr. Leonidas Berry, Advisory Commission member, clinical professor at the University of Illinois and practicing physician, predicted at the first meeting of the Commission: "Probably the most difficult area in developing cooperative arrangements will be that which projects the interface between medical center professionals and community-based practicing physicians."[20]

Medical schools were indeed to be at the center of the arrangements. But from the beginning there was an expectation that, though it might take considerable time, the more organizations, institutions, and professionals included in the cooperative arrangements, the better. There were two more things: cooperative arrangements were to have an identifiable, responsible administrative structure, plus advisory councils; and the aggregate activity of regional medical programs should add up to more than a series of diverse projects.

The general exhortation for health professionals and health care delivery institutions to cooperate would have been unlikely to stir action had not some millions of dollars been offered to support this proposed cooperation, $55 million being authorized for the first year. And so, for the first time, in 55 self-delineated regions of the country, medical school deans, hospital administrators, medical society officers and representatives of professional associations and state agencies did in fact come together to create such programs. They did so in a variety of ways and with a variety of structures. They even did so, despite the first categorical emphases of the legislation, with a variety of priorities, often but not always beginning with heart disease, cancer and stroke.

These various arrangements will be described in the chapters that follow, but it is not too soon to report that the most striking and consistent features among Regional Medical Programs in the ten years of their formal existence were patterns of creative partnerships, of information sharing and sometimes resource sharing, and of occasional unified purpose and operation. This practice was exactly what the originators of the program, from LBJ to Mike DeBakey to several Surgeons General, and several directors of the Division of Regional Programs, devoutly hoped would occur.

Notes:

1. U.S. Department of Health, Education, and Welfare, "Proceedings: Conferences on Regional Medical Programs," June, 1967, p. 40.
2. David A. Pearson "The Concept of Regionalized Personal Health Services in the United States, 1920, 1955," in The Regionalization of Personal Health Services, Ernest W., M.D. (Ed.) (New York: Milbank Memorial Fund, 1975) pp. 5-10.
3. Ibid., pp. 10-11.
4. William Kissick, M.D., Regionalization of U.S. Health Care, manuscript in progress, Chapter 6, 1993.
5. Ibid.
6. Ibid.
7. U.S. Congress, Senate Committee on Education and Labor, "Hearings on Wartime Health and Education," 78th Congress., 2nd session, 2, Jan. 1945, pp. 2196-2198.
8. Hearings, op. cit. See discussion in Stephen P. Strickland, Politics, Science and Dread Disease, (Cambridge, Mass: Harvard University Press, 1972) Chapter II. See also discussions in Pearson, op. cit., pp.18-19, 26-32.

9. Hearings, op. cit.

10. Ibid.

11. U.S.D.H.E.W., 1967 Conference Proceedings, op. cit., p 113.

12. Op. cit., p. 40.

13. Interview with Karl Yordy.

14. Public Law 89-749, 89th Congress.

15. Strickland, op. cit., p. 209.

16. Public Law 89-239, 89th Congress, 3.596, Oct. 8, 1965, Title IX, Sec. 900 (a).

17. U. S. Congress, Committee on Interstate and Foreign Commerce, House Report 963, accompanying H.R. 3140, 89th Congress; U.S.D.H.E.W., Division of Regional Medical Programs, NIH, "Guidelines for Regional Medical Programs," July 1966.

18. Public Law 89-239, op. cit., Title IX, Sec 900 (b).

19. Leonidas K. Berry, M.D., "Development of Cooperative Arrangements for Regional Medical Programs," Remarks at Conference on Regional medical Programs. January 1967, Washington, DC, Papers of Dr. Berry, RMP Archives of the National Library of Medicine.

Chapter 5

Regional Medical Programs Take Shape

Despite the challenges of definition and delineation, within six months after the publication of guidelines for Regional Medical Programs in July of 1966, fifty-four regions had organized themselves. Fifty of those had been given planning grants by the Surgeon General following the approval of the National Advisory Council.[1]

New York

The Albany (New York) Regional Medical Program was the first one in the nation to be approved, in January 1966. Encompassing the city of Albany, twenty-one surrounding counties in New York, a bit of southern New Hampshire and Brooklyn County in Massachusetts, the region was to serve a population of approximately 2 million persons. There were eighty-seven hospitals in the region thus delineated. The Albany College of Medicine of Union University assumed the leadership in organizing the region and the program.[2]

The State of New York was ultimately to have six regional programs based within it. In October 1966, the Rochester RNP was formed, centered in that city but serving ten surrounding counties and 1.3 million people.[3] In January 1967, one year after Albany, the Central New York RMP was awarded a planning grant; this program centered on Syracuse and was to serve fifteen counties in the State of New York plus two in Pennsylvania, with a total population of little less than two million persons.[4] Buffalo and the Lakes Area came next and Long Island -- Nassau and Suffolk Counties — followed much later.[5]

What happened in New York City was a demonstration of the difficulties of organizing a large metropolitan area into a region, developing cooperative arrangements within it for the identification of medical needs and coordinating the resources needed to meet them.[6] Delineating the territory turned out to be the easiest job. The New York Regional Medical Program included the five boroughs of New York City plus four counties: Westchester, Orange, Rockland, and Putnam. The total population to be served was almost nine million people, seven million of whom lived in New York City. All medical schools in the city -- Cornell, Columbia, New York Medical School, and New York University School of Medicine -- were directly involved in the early stages of the organization. All sent representatives to the early meetings, as did, occasionally, the Downstate Medical School in Stoneybrook, Long Island. Scores of hospitals were involved, particularly those affiliated with the medical schools. The medical schools were relatively large and, except for Downstate, were private. Through their affiliated teaching hospitals each had some connections (though not necessarily strong ones) with adjacent communities and with the New York City population generally.

The medical schools were research institutions as well as teaching institutions. Columbia, NYU and Cornell were known for faculties whose expertise was such that they received substantial quantities of biomedical research grants from the National Institutes of Health. Regional Medical Programs, being authorized at the level of $50 million for the first year, in contrast to the NIH appropriation of $1 billion, must have seemed like small potatoes.

"However, most schools did not want to see another get ahead with the RMP business," recalled Dr. George Reader, who represented Cornell on the New York Metropolitan RMP Council. The arrangement decided upon was to locate the coordinating body in the New York Academy of Medicine. The Academy was willing to serve this purpose, but, as Dr. Reader remembers it, placing it there "did not accomplish much" since its traditional focus was on education and it had no capacity for delivery of services.[7]

But while the medical schools did not want to lose out in any competition for RMP funds or glory, neither were they greatly enthusiastic about the program: "Cornell was less than enthusiastic about RMP's stated objective of bringing new techniques to the bedside... Most of the effort went into extending programs already in place."[8]

When Dr. Reader was chosen as Cornell's representative on the advisory council, he was enthusiastic. So was the President of the New York Hospital-Cornell Medical Center, Dr. Joe Hennesey. But Cornell's Dean certainly did not have time to get involved. Nor did any other medical school dean take an active role. So, at Cornell, Dr. Reeder, the Chairman of the Department of Public Health, was sent to do the job. He found others in similar positions in their respective schools also there; some of them were more and some less interested in about RMP. In general, there was "a remarkable lack of enthusiasm in the rest of the New York medical community about all of this."[9]   Indeed, what interest there was seemed to be at two levels. The president of the Academy was very positive, as was the Commissioner of Health in New York, Dr. George James. But Dr. James was shortly asked to be President of a new medical school, Mt. Sinai, and was so consumed in that awesome challenge that he had little time for the new RMP that he had publicly boosted..

Not that the idea of regionalization would fall completely by the wayside.   Dr. James' successor as Health Commissioner, Mary McLaughlin, thought that every hospital in the city should have a region, a geographical area within the city, it could focus on. Some of the hospitals made an effort at this but an early survey showed that many New Yorkers got their medical care from facilities, including emergency rooms, nearest to their subway lines, not necessarily to their residences.[10] Two years after the New York Metropolitan RMP received its planning grant, it still had not presented program plans and requests to fund them to the National Advisory Council on Regional Medical Programs. In mid-1969, it still had not received funds to support programs.[11]

Meanwhile, Albany, with its smaller geographical region and population, with all medical education centered at Albany Medical College, and with the history of local "regionalism," began funding projects that were part of an overall plan approved by the National Advisory Council on April 1, 1967.[12] Continuing education was a principal emphasis, one of the first projects being to identify professional education needs of physicians in the region and develop a program to respond to them. In order to build continuing dialogue and cooperation among various health professionals who were to be involved in his program, Albany quickly created a special team to ensure such interaction. Four former pharmaceutical company representatives were engaged by Albany "to evaluate the liaison, evaluate prevailing attitudes, and promote effective personal contact and lay individuals and groups who have a role in the developing Regional Medical Program."[13] Several coronary care demonstration programs were designated for support. The two-way radio communication system already in place in a dozen hospitals was expanded to an additional fifty-seven.

By July 1968, the Central New York RMP was up and running. Centered at the Upstate Medical Center, it promptly appointed committees to deal with heart disease, cancer and stroke. Its first project efforts were in these areas, with special emphasis on updating nursing skills in each of them.[14] In Central New York's case, as in many other regional programs developing across the country, the principal activity was in continuing medical education.[15] This was natural because it was that component part of the problem of delivering the latest advances in medical care to people all over the country -- despite the protestation of some that there was no lag -- that had been the original impetus of the national program. Further, as was observed in the course of the January 1967 national review in Washington: "Many of the participants were willing, even eager, to settle most of the efforts, funds, and hopes for the regional medical program concept on this one area, which both the medical education establishment and practitioners readily agree is important and essentially non-threatening to existing patterns of the delivery of health services."[16]

The varying success, or lack of it, among the programs located within in the State of New York was illustrative of a pattern that would occur throughout the country.

Illinois

Medical health leaders in eastern Illinois made serious if gradual, comprehensive if cautious attempts to organize a regional medical program that would serve the entire state.[17] It was to be centered in Chicago, but it was to include the deans of the five Illinois medical schools, plus the College of Osteopathy, and the heads of their major teaching hospitals. It also included the leadership of the Illinois State

Medical Society, the Chicago Medical Society, the Illinois Hospital Association, the Illinois Department of Public Health, and the Hospital Planning Council of Metropolitan Chicago among others. With the Chairman, Dr. Oglesby Paul from Northwestern University School of Medicine and the Program Coordinator, Dr. Wright Adams from University of Chicago Pritzger School of Medicine, the organizing committee secured its planning grant in July 1967. The program next succeeded in including leaders from the Illinois Division of the American Cancer Society and the Chicago and Illinois Heart Associations.

The official governing group and its state entity associates "felt that the state boundaries would constitute the best region, for certainly the Illinois Regional Medical Program interest is statewide."[18] They acknowledged that "persons living in communities nearest the state borders do not allow political lines to limit them as they seek health care."[19] This meant that Illinois RMP would perhaps pay attention to communities across state borders; that "major regions centered in large metropolitan areas may well undergo a subregional development facing their apex upon smaller yet fully qualified areas;"[20] and that IRMP would cooperate with other regional medical programs in adjacent states and regions. This approach was a sensible one philosophically and practically. For one thing the Bi-State program, centered in St. Louis with eastern Missouri and southern Illinois in its purview, was already operating.

The Illinois program otherwise gradually became established in all other parts of the state. Given the mere size of Illinois -- with its approximately 9 million persons, almost all to be served by IRNP -- its combination of urban and rural populations, and the number of medical schools and major health care providing agencies of institutions, this program also did not submit a plan for operations until 1969, after the law had been extended for another two years. But the reasons for this were different from those that obtained in Metropolitan New York.

Connecticut

Whereas in some states and metropolitan areas the elements were regional cooperation were already in place when the national program created by the Heart Disease, Cancer and Stroke Amendments of 1965 became operational, in other places they were not. Connecticut was one of the latter.

Indeed, in some ways, despite the geographic smallness of the State and a population of only 3 million people, health care was a very fractionated matter. The Yale University School of Medicine had been the dominant medical institution in image, and in some ways in reality, for as long as anyone could remember. That is, until the creation of a School of Medicine at the University of Connecticut in Farmington just a few years before the Regional Medical Programs began. Even at Yale, members of the medical faculty were not often in contact with the faculty at the School of Public Health, though it was one of the oldest, most active and most distinguished such school in the country. The School of Medicine could realistically claim to be a national institution, in terms of its student body, its rank in medical education and medical research, and in its faculty. Yale was not, in short, particularly focused on or concerned about the population of Connecticut.[21]

There were plenty of practicing physicians in the State. Despite the typical concentration of them in cities -- Hartford, New Haven, Bridgeport -- the maldistribution problem which plagued the country generally and some states dramatically was not a major factor within the borders of Connecticut.

In the early months of Regional Medical Programs, the only alliance which came together was that of the two medical schools which actually began regular communication because of the new program. Yale, the old, distinguished institution was the first grantee agency for CRMP, putting together a plan that secured its first grant from the national program to begin activities on July 1, 1966. In October of that year, Dr. Henry T. Clark Jr. joined as the first the first director of the program. One of the things that must have won him favor from those making the selection was his involvement years before in the Rochester, New York area where metropolitan regionalism had a strong and successful history. He had also, in Puerto Rico a decade before, secured the agreement of 16 local committees in the eastern part of the Commonwealth to create an integrated medical care network, a pattern of consultative and cooperative planning leading to action which was most unusual in the health care scene across America.

Dr. Clark urged Connecticut to move carefully and analytically.

Shortly after his arrival, "we launched an 18- month study of the health delivery system of Connecticut, under the aegis of nine representative state-wide task forces supported by research personnel from the Yale University School of Public Health."[22] Such studies are not so unusual; indeed the value of them has always seemed self-evident especially when, as in the case of Lyndon Johnson's original impulse, there already exists a predilection to do something. But the Connecticut study's purpose was not just to determine strengths and weaknesses in the aggregate health care picture of the State but "to get the necessary consensus among providers."[23]

The consensus focused on fundamentals. Connecticut was almost naturally divided into "ten health service areas."[24] The general hospitals in each area were "encouraged to work together." All of the general hospitals not already affiliated with the Yale or Connecticut Schools of Medicine were encouraged to do so. The encouragement was concrete: CRMP would pay part of the salaries of newly appointed full-time hospital Chiefs of Service in various medical specialties, who would also have clinical faculty appointments at one of the two medical schools.[25]

Yale's sphere of influence was in the eastern part of the state. The University of Connecticut's was in the west. CRMP also supported an Office for Continuing Education to coordinate planning among the various agencies, including private associations such as the Heart Association and the Cancer Society, which already sponsored continuing education. It provided financial and technical assistance for local long-range planning within the ten health service areas of the region. CRMP provided the two university medical center libraries with additional personnel and equipment; it paid for programs that linked these two medical libraries to those in the ten areas.

According to Dr. John Thompson of the Yale University School of Public Health and a member of the National Advisory Council of RMP, "the Connecticut Program studied everything."[26] It supported studies of patterns of organization of services; comparative studies of mobile coronary care units and multiplication of such units in community hospitals; studies on financing of institutional medical care (including "analyses of capital funding, cash flow, reimbursement formulae of third party agents, and the rate of self-paid patients"); and studies of studies including "feasibility studies related to design of long-range evaluation."

The first comprehensive study was that which was the basis for the Connecticut plan. Although this took a year and a half, by July 1, 1969, the Connecticut Regional Medical Program was established. It was an organization officially separate from Yale and the University of Connecticut, governed by a "Board of Directors or Trustees... made up of 36 members, and covering the whole gamut of health interests in the state ...[27]

As the 1970's began, Connecticut could point to specific advances, at least in the system. Twenty-nine of the thirty-three general hospitals in the state were by then affiliated with one of the two medical schools; almost as many for the first time had appointed full-time Chiefs of Service. Dr. George Silver, back in Connecticut after a long stint in top policy circles in Washington, remembers that there was consensus that the hospitals in Bridgeport, Danbury, and Waterbury were on their way to becoming first-rate. Patterns of cooperation in the ten regions could be identified, especially in terms in the treatment of heart disease and cancer.

Yet as Dr. Clark straightforwardly acknowledged in 1973, five years after he began his tour of duty as the CRMP's director, there remained a central need and challenge. He wrote: "There is a desperate need for various parts of the health establishment -- i.e. the practicing professions, the university health centers, the general hospitals and long-term care institutions, the public agencies such as the Departments of Public Health, Mental Health and Welfare, and a host of voluntary agencies -- to work together to solve present problems of health care delivery..."[28] He was talking both about the nation generally and about Connecticut. Regionalization of medical services was "the best hope for putting needed order in our health care delivery system."[29] General cooperative arrangements such as those he and his colleagues had finally been able to put in place in the State were tantamount to "a tiny patch of blue" in an otherwise dismal sky.[30]

What was really needed -- after the Connecticut legislature activated a new commission to perform the requisite study -- was a formal program of medical regionalization for the State, each governed by a health care authority. The study commission was to decide how much authority the health care agencies should have, but it was clearly more than the Regional Medical Program had. For only real authority, in contrast to the general charge to encourage cooperative arrangements, could produce the "needed order in our health care delivery system."[31]

Notes:

1. U.S. Department of Health, Education and Welfare, Division of Regional Medical Programs, "Directory of Regional Medical Programs." 1969, p.
2. Ibid.
3. Ibid.
4. Ibid.
5. Ibid.
6. Some details of descriptions of the Metropolitan New York RMP are taken from "Directory of Regional Medical Programs," op. cit. The central story comes principally from an interview with Dr. George Reader who represented Cornell Medical School in both the organizing committee and subsequently the Regional Advisory Group for the duration of the program. Interview conducted in New York on Dr. Reader's last day as a faculty member at Cornell, before his retirement, on June 30, 1992. Additional details provided in a letter from Dr. Reader to Dr. Donald Lindberg, Dec. 11, 1991.
7. Interview.
8. Ibid.
9. Ibid.
10. Ibid.
11. "Directory of Regional Medical Programs," op. cit.
12. Frank M. Woolsey, Jr., "Albany Emphasizes Community Strength, Relationships," Albany Medical College Bulletin, 1969.
13. Ibid., p.4.
14. "Directory of Regional Medical Programs, op. cit.
15. See "The RMP Experience: Nine Years of Working with Local People to Improve Health Care," Central New York Regional Medical Program, Final Report, Sept. 1976.
16. U.S. DHEW, "Proceedings: Conference on Regional Medical Programs," January 15-17, 1967, p.64.
17. Wright Adams, 11 The Illinois Regional Medical Program for Heart Disease, Cancer and Stroke," Illinois Medical Journal, Feb. 1969.
18. Ibid., p.167.
19. Ibid.
20. Ibid.
21. Interviews with Dr. John Thompson and Dr. George Silver, July 8-9, 1992. See also Connecticut Regional Medical Program, "CRMP's Seven Year March toward Medical Regionalization," March 1973.
22. Henry T. Clark, Jr., "The Connecticut Regional Medical Program," Connecticut Medical Journal June 1973.
23. Ibid.
24. Edward F. Morrisey, Conrad Seipp, and Henry T. Clark, Jr., "Connecticut

50

Regional Medical Program - From Planning to Operations," Connecticut Medicine, Feb. 1969, p.108. See also E. Richard Weikerman, "Planning and Organization of the Connecticut Regional Medical Program," Bulletin of the New York Academy of Medicine, June 1969.

25. Morrisey, Seipp and Clark, op. cit.
26. Interview with Dr. Thompson.
27. "Connecticut Regional Medical Program - From Planning to Operations" op. cit., p. 112.
28. Henry T. Clark, "Connecticut Regional Medical Program: Health Care Planning," Connecticut Medicine, Jan. 1973, p.33.
29. Ibid.
30. Ibid., p. 34.
31. Ibid.

Chapter 6

North Carolina

Before the ink was dry on the Heart Disease, Cancer and Stroke Amendments of 1965, the Executive Council of the Medical Society of the State of North Carolina responded by creating a ten-member advisory council of health professionals. This council represented the three medical schools existing in the state -- Duke, University of North Carolina, and Bowman-Gray -- the State Board of Health, the Medical Care Commission, the medical society itself, and a number of hospitals. Over the next several months, the council did an informal survey of resources and needs, especially with respect to the principal disease categories emphasized in the new federal act, and with respect to continuing education for various health professions vis à vis these needs. In April 1966, with program plans barely organized and articulated at the national level, the State Advisory Council applied for recognition of the North Carolina Regional Medical Program and created a non-profit association to be administrator of the program. To the medical schools and other institutions already involved was added the University of North Carolina School of Public Health. The advisory council then became the Board of Directors of the association.[1]

Sixteen months later, in October of 1967, North Carolina Regional Medical Program submitted a request for operational funds to the national program, both for the administration of the program and for a number of projects.[2]   The North Carolina program was awarded almost $1.5 million. One of the first projects was to establish a network of coronary care units in small community hospitals in the western part of the state; a parallel one was to develop a system of consultation services for coronary care training and development. There was begun a central cancer registry and cancer information service, and a state-wide network of ambulances equipped with the technology and trained personnel to provide immediate care of acute coronary attacks at the site where they occurred. Almost all program bases were touched. There was a diabetes program, one on continuing education in internal medicine, another on continuing education of dentists.[3] There was a joint effort of the three medical schools to combine the facilities and talents of those working in their respective libraries, "to extend, in a meaningful way, a giant educational service to all practicing physicians in the state."[4]

This sequence of events, summed up in early 1968 by Mark J. Musser, M.D., Executive Director of the NCRMP, was the result of an extraordinary series of conversations among principal health care providers, educators and policy makers in the particular regions during this period. For the first time in memory, the deans of North Carolina's three medical schools sat down with leaders of the Medical Society and the State Board of Health and talked about how a regional medical program might strengthen their individual as well as their combined capacities to deliver medical care. RMP was not seen as the be- all, end-all approach to obvious problems. But it was seen -- even before the final version was passed by Congress and signed by the President and guidelines formed by the national organization -- as "one vehicle by means of which the medical schools can logically and effectively participate in revising our system for delivery of health sciences; and participate we must."[5]

The details of those early conversations are fascinating, and the spirit striking.[6] One element leaps out of interview notes and other records: In that remarkable period of policy expansion and social and political activism of a national administration, the mere proposal of a new federally supported program of regional partnerships to serve people was enough to inspire intellectual and action-oriented ferment in communities, regions, and states. Vice President Al Gore in early 1994 asserted that the mere existence of a formal national health plan by the Clinton administration was precipitating changes for the better in the financing system. Whether or not that assessment has held up over the past five years, after the sinking of the Clinton health plan, is not clear. Nonetheless, the syndrome pointed out by Gore was definitely at work in North Carolina and elsewhere in 1965 as President Johnson and his commission proposed new strategies, and as the Congress and principally affected groups such as the American Medical Association and the Association of American Medical Colleges reacted to them.

The conversations among the medical school deans and other North Carolina power figures are confirmed by persons who were present and others who benefitted from their legacy. In the ensuing months and years, as RMP was formally being organized, the medical schools continued their conversations. Early in the program's development, the deans agreed on a strategy which would permit each school to serve delineated geographical areas and constituencies, some already being served and others theretofore unreached. Together the schools would fill in gaps -- both in the eastern and western parts of the state where there were, at that point, no medical schools -- through joint programs.

There was also sub-regional ferment. The seven counties of the westernmost part of the state resurrected a term stemming from the Civil War years, when some of those counties tried to secede from North Carolina after it had seceded from the Union, and assert the independence of the State of Franklin. This time, the notion was not secession, but strengthening links within that region, so that the new "State of Franklin" would be prepared to cooperate with the North Carolina Regional Medical Program and receive the most benefit from it. This arrangement, which may seem natural and normal, was nonetheless quite a stretch for the independent-minded inhabitants of the separate county jurisdictions and the municipalities within them. And it both shored up strengths and exposed weaknesses in health care provision which have lasted to this day.[7]

The North Carolina experience, like others examples reported in this study, reminds us once again that there are two basic elements to any successful human endeavor, the institutional and the human. The state plan, as it was gradually and steadily developed in cooperative fashion, was to cover the state using the expertise of particular institutions and other entities, and to do so on the basis of established political boundaries, natural constituencies, and utilization of institutional and professional strengths within each. The grid through which the combined forces would work was a composite of nine geographical areas, at the center of which -- in thinking and planning -- was a program of continuing education of physicians, nurses and other health professionals.

The origins of these developments date back began before the advent of Great Society health legislation. They even antedate the general concern about clinical training and geographic distribution of health manpower that reached its zenith in the early seventies. For example, some of the impetus for the North Carolina Area Health Education Centers occurred in the early 1940's when the University of North Carolina School of Medicine at Chapel Hill expanded to a four-year program and adopted a de facto mandate to help meet the physician manpower needs of the state.[8] In the early 1960's the School began to explore ways of decentralizing the clinical education of the students and in that connection, developed affiliations with community hospitals to provide clinical training for those students. In 1965 the UNC Medical School formally created a division of education and research in community medical care to oversee this program and related activities.

Then with Regional Medical Programs looming as an imminent possibility in 1965, the three schools joined together to support similar extensions of the training. It is not unfair to describe the planning, and programs that developed from it, as centrally if collaboratively directed. The community institutions and regional arrangements (e.g., the State of Franklin) contributed to an interaction, created a synergy that surely must have pleased the President of the United States and all those who worked with him to shape Regional Medical Programs.

Then as now, states and their actions did not always prove the inherent virtue of federalism. They were, then as now, often battlegrounds in which mayors and others representing their urban constituencies carried out direct and indirect battle with powerful legislators from rural areas, representing theirs. There were struggles between those who thought state government should reduce its role vis a vis health and welfare, and those who thought the state must take the lead in these areas with or without federal support. There were partisan divisions and professional divisions; there were geographical divisions and divisions along scores of other axes. Still, given what is often a mythic sense of common bond and history as well as a focused constitutional authority, in many instances it was fundamentally a "sense of state" that inspired, and occasionally even galvanized, citizens and communities into action.

This is not the place for a long discussion of state pride. But state pride had much to do with the collaboration of the North Carolina medical deans in forging a new partnership in the mid-sixties, and the state medical societies in endorsing and facilitating it. Those surveying the state landscape from the "ivory towers" of Duke, Wake Forest and UNC saw clearly the needs of people far removed from them. Except for this vision of and commitment to their state, they might have remained in their own worlds, unattached and uninvolved, and the North Carolina Regional Medical Program might have been undistinguished and unimportant.

The sense of pride in state, often clear-eyed and coupled with recognition of serious problems, is not unique to North Carolina. But the spirit of North Carolinians and their leaders in the public and private sector has to be related to the enormous strides that state has made in the past three decades in education and commerce and in myriad other ways. It was clearly an important factor in the creation and continuation of the North Carolina Regional Medical Program.

There are dozens of successful examples of medical programs begun with the help of RMP. The diabetes program begun by an interested UNC faculty member and involving the several medical schools and a number of community hospitals, actually spurred the creation of a state-wide diabetes association -- a reversal of the more typical situation of an "interest group" pushing for the creation of a responsible program.[9]

Area Health Education Centers are a special case. The North Carolina AHEC program benefitted significantly from early RMP support. Then, in 1974 when federal manpower support funds, including those provided through Regional Medical Programs and through the Bureau of Health Manpower Education in Washington, were already beginning to decline, the North Carolina General Assembly appropriated $28.2 million dollars to strengthen and expand the programs as part of a state-wide plan for health professional education.[10] Even though fiscal times have been lean in recent years, the people of the state, the charitable foundations and the state government continue to believe in regional programs at least in the form in which North Carolina has carried them. In September 1998, North Carolina's AHEC program reached its silver anniversary in golden form.

56

Notes:

1. Marc J. Musser, M.D., "The Regional Medical Program in North Carolina," North Carolina Medical Journal, June 1968, p.240.
2. Ibid.
3. Ibid., pp. 240-241.
4. Ibid., p. 241. S. Ibid.
5. Other sources for this chapter come from interviews in April 1993 conducted by the author with several persons involved in the creation of the North Carolina Regional Medical Program including: Dr. Harvey Estes, North Carolina Medical Society Foundation; Dr. Eugene Mayer, now Associate Dean of the University of North Carolina School of Medicine and AHEC Program Director; James Bernstein, Director, N.C. Office of Rural Health and Resource Development; and Dr. Clarence Scheps, Distinguished Professor of Social Medicine Emeritus and former department head at the University of North Carolina School of Medicine. Other resources include an interview conducted by Diane Rehm with Dr. T. Franklin Williams, July 26, 1991, at the National Library of Medicine.
6. See Ralph S. Morgan, M.D., "Development of a Regional Medical Program in Western North Carolina," North Carolina Medical Journal, May 1967, 195-197 passim.
7. "1991 Progress Report," North Carolina Area Health Education Centers Program, University of North Carolina at Chapel Hill. See also Rebecca W. Davidson, "The Library/Learning Resource Center Network of the North Carolina AHEC Program," UNC Health Sciences Library, August 28, 1991. Introduction and Chronology, VI - X.
8. T. Franklin Williams, M.D., Interview conducted by Diane Rehm, July 1991, NLM, pp. 1-2.
9. Davidson, op. cit., P.VIII.

Chapter 7

Georgia and Florida: Study in Contrasts

In January 1966 the Georgia Advisory Group for the Regional Medical Program got underway, with the assistance of representatives from the Medical Association of Georgia as well as from the dental, pharmaceutical, hospital and nurses associations of the State; from the Georgia Heart Association and the Georgia Division of the American Cancer Society and from the Emory University School of Medicine and the Medical College of Georgia. Dr. J. Willis Hurst, a member of the DeBakey Commission and the National Advisory Council for Regional Medical Programs, served as chairman of the steering committee of the GRMP. In the latter role, Dr. Hurst was instrumental in writing the planning grant application for the Georgia program which was submitted in September of 1966 and approved by the Surgeon General in December.[1] Dr. Hurst asked an Emory School colleague, Dr. J. Gordon Barrow, a clinical professor of medicine in cardiology and private practitioner at George Baptist Hospital, to become the Director on the Georgia Program.

Emory shared with the Medical College of Georgia the role of educating the state's physicians. It was estimated that 80% of the doctors practicing in Georgia had graduated from either Emory or the Medical College of Georgia.[2] This meant that, as a general proposition, there was relatively easy communication between the medical schools and medical associations, and equally important, between the general and community hospitals around the state and the two medical schools. But there was competition as well as communication between the two schools. This produced an interesting result when the Georgia Regional Medical Program was getting underway. The Medical Association of Georgia supported the new program and was to take an extremely active part in organizing and implementing it. In fact, the MAG offered to be the grant recipient for the program and provide space for its headquarters in Atlanta for Dr. Barrow and the RMP staff.

A key reason for the Association's interest in becoming the grantee agency and exercise a little oversight was, according to Dr. Barrow, that the practicing physicians "just wanted to make sure that in Georgia, RMP didn't funnel money into the medical schools just for medical school purposes.... They wanted it to be a community program to strengthen medicine in the community, because they understood that improving the care for heart disease, cancer and stroke was what it was all about."[3]

Georgia is the second largest state in size (after Pennsylvania) east of the Mississippi River. It has 150 counties and, in 1966, had scores of county and multi-county medical societies. Atlanta and Augusta, with their respective medical schools and affiliated hospitals, were the centers of medical sophistication in the State. Overall there were more than 175 general hospitals across Georgia, with three thousand physicians serving on their staffs.[4]

So that the Georgia program would reach all medical and health professionals delivering care, and through them the people of the state, the advisory group proposed a plan to create intra-state regions; each would have a principal hospital as the focal point and each an advisory group. The concrete objective was that every hospital would become an adequate teaching hospital. That was a tall order for some communities, but Dr. Hurst and his colleagues were quick to explain: "This does not imply that medical students, interns and residents need to be present" in each hospital. "It does imply the physicians, nurses, dentists, members of the public and all the allied health professions" -- including nurses aids, technicians, dietitians, psychologists, physical, occupational, and speech therapists, social workers and "all others are now or may be in the future related to the care of patients" -- shall organize themselves into an educational program."[5]

There were certain details to be worked out. Obviously, some cities in the State of Georgia had more than one hospital. The advisory group simply acknowledged, in its application for a planning grant, that "it would be necessary to study the activities of each of these hospitals... to develop a working relationship of each hospital with the other."[6] The plan envisioned a system that connected the two medical schools and certain larger hospitals in the state to the smaller hospitals. Communication among the subregions, and between them and the program staff and advisory group, was the key operational element. It was agreed that the chairman of the local groups would come together at least twice a year to compare experience and plans; and it was very soon decided that the staff should include field representatives, five in all, who would be the active day-to-day communication links between the program headquarters in Atlanta and the State at large. The representatives were not medical professionals. "But most of them were young college-educated men with an interest in traveling over the State... they just traveled and talked RMP, is what it amounted to. They were communication people." [7]

The planning grant proposal even suggested how the local advisory groups were to be organized. A hospital administrator, a physician, a nurse and an interested member of the public were the minimum number of people selected to represent the hospital. "These individuals will be named through acceptable administrative mechanisms. For example, the physician would be selected by the hospital staff and serve as chairman of the group; the administrator would be selected by the administrators of the hospitals; the nurse would be selected by the organized nursing service, or if such is not present, would be selected by the hospital administrator acting jointly with the hospital staff. The member of the public would be selected by the hospital governing board; and others in local official and non-official health agencies may be asked to serve." [8]

The whole point of the local advisory groups was that each would serve both "as a nucleus to stimulate a new interest in continuing education, a new consciousness of community health problems, and a new curiosity to evaluate, appraise and measure the effectiveness of our present day approach to the problems of stroke heart disease, cancer and other related diseases." [9]

Within six months, on June 4, 1967, the Georgia Regional Medical Program had called a meeting in Atlanta. Eighty-eight advisory group chairmen and others representing 79 community hospitals already signed up to participate were in attendance. The meeting was opened by Dr. John Malden, President of the Medical Association of Georgia. Dr. William

Mayer, Associate Director of the Division of Regional Programs of NIH, was on hand to elaborate overall purposes and guidelines and to answer questions. He was praised for "his ability to make the complex law clear to everyone." [10]

The meeting was an obvious attempt to stir enthusiasm and organizational support, and it seems to have done just that. Within weeks, the steering committee of the Georgia RMP had organized disease-oriented task forces and coordinating units looking at suggested needs in health manpower, continuing education in libraries, hospital facilities, and epidemiology. The higher system was viewed as both "a university without walls" and as a cooperative arrangement among all the physicians and other health professionals, medical schools and hospitals organized for the purpose of "giving better care to our patients." [11]

The Georgia Medical Association, the black doctors' counterpart organization to the MAG, was invited to participate and soon became an important partner. For example, it played an important role in developing hypertension screening programs over the next decade.

The ambition of the Georgia Plan was comprehensive and specific. Dr. Barrow recalls that one of the ideas was "to create medical centers within 30 or 40 miles of everybody within the State that would be able to treat heart disease, cancer and stroke in a first-class manner." [12] And regardless of the national controversy in medical association circles about the DeBakey Commission's phrase, the Georgians decided to support the development of "medical centers of excellence" built around major hospitals. This meant that, in addition to Atlanta and Augusta, there would be centers in Thomasville, Albany, Valdosta, Savannah, Brunswick, Macon, Rome, Gainesville, and a couple of others cities and towns. In addition, there would be a series of "health access stations," located in rural areas in which either there was no physician or a gross shortage of physicians, and as well, in urban low-income areas where easy accessibility to a physician was a problem. [13]

> The health access station was to serve five basic purposes: 1) to provide emergency first aid when needed; 2) to provide transportation, if needed, to and from the physician or nearby hospital; 3) to assist the patient who does not have a physician to obtain one; 4) to assist the physician in the assessment of clinical condition of the remote patient (apparently with the first examination by a nurse or physicians assistant); 5) to assist the physician in the follow-up

of his patient and to assist the patient in carrying out the physicians instructions.[14]

Dr. Barrow stated the preface to and premise for the access stations as follows: "Doctors of the state are beginning to realize that medical care is considered by most to be the right of all citizens and, if the profession does not solve the problem of accessibility and availability of care in areas in where it is deficient, the state or federal government will probably take steps to solve it." [15] He and his colleagues invited doctors to participate in the system of health access stations. The response was good. Dr. Barrow subsequently reported that five such stations were established in the first year each with registered nurses on duty.

Records of the clinics kept on a weekly basis showed that by 1972, an average of 100 to 200 patients per month were being seen at each station. The records revealed that the stations were being utilized by both black and white patients; that adults and children were being served in patterns proportionate to the population; and that female use predominated over male. [16] Dr. Barrow asserted that both the public and area physicians were generally enthusiastic about the system. He noted that the enthusiasm among doctors was especially strong where the local health access station was sponsored by the local medical society.

Simultaneously, the Georgia Program set about setting up cancer, stroke and heart clinics all over the state, free of charge for those that could not afford to pay. In the next several years, approximately sixteen programs were established, with RMP paying the salaries of the nurses in charge and, in some instances, paying for the space. But many of the clinics were housed in local hospitals which provided the utilities and in some cases the space itself. Indeed, "the hospitals supported this so strongly that if you were going to be on the medical staff... you had to give a certain amount of time to these free clinics." [17]

There seems to have been no significant opposition to the health access stations or clinics on the part of organized medicine. The provision of free medical care by doctors to patients in need is, of course, a part of the professional ethic and tradition. In Georgia, "Before RMP came along, a lot of doctors were seeing patients in their offices and not charging them because they knew they were poor and couldn't pay." They were also doing it because the doctors who referred them also referred their paying patients. Naturally "they didn't want to hurt that doctor's feelings." [18] When such patients "could be handled in a clinic, it was so much cheaper on the doctor. It didn't take near as much time as it did in his own office. So it cost him less to participate in the clinic and see the patients there." The Georgia Program charged all patients who came to the access stations or clinics a minimal charge, a dollar per visit in the case of the access stations. [19]

The Georgia Regional Medical Program was receiving $1-2 million when the program was fully operative, and spent an estimated total of $25 million over the decade. Within that decade, hypertension rates in the state had been reduced. The continuing education program envisioned at the outset had been realized. Most Georgians were within 50 miles from a doctor and a nurse who dispensed care and made referrals, working for free or for modest fees paid by the Regional Medical Program. Subregional hospitals become more sophisticated in their capacities.

More people with heart disease, cancer and stroke, renal disease and diabetes were being treated. Twenty hospitals had developed their cancer diagnostic capacities and in some cases their capacity to treat cancer. There had been a significant expansion of the number of cardiac care units in Georgia, with RMP paying for the training of several hundred nurses and physicians in charge of the units in the first two years of the program.

When the Georgia Regional Medical Program was terminated in October 1976, Dr. Barrow reported that out of its aggregate ten-year budget, grants totaling more than $18 million had been made to Georgia institutions and health related agencies. A significant part of these funds were spent in medical schools. The Medical Association of Georgia had also received some funds, more than $600,000 for the space it had provided GRMP in its building for 10 years and project grants totalling about $285,000. Also during the decade, "the county societies and foundations associated with the Medical Association have received grants totaling $175,775.13." [20]

All those involved believed, with Dr. Barrow, that the "leadership provided by the medical community and the activities of the Regional Medical Programs have resulted in one of the outstanding programs of health services development in the country." As he ended his tour of duty,

Dr. Barrow received special recognition from the dean and faculty of Emory School of Medicine: "Through his leadership he has brought great honor to the program and the people in this State." [21]

Florida

While the Medical Association of Georgia was enthusiastically embracing Regional Medical Programs, the Medical Society of Florida was having a fit. Or at least it was having great difficulty coming to terms with the proposed new national plan. It was no doubt more difficult to organize that elongated state with its diverse population (and in 1965 with three medical schools) than other Southern states. But it is noteworthy that it took almost two years longer for the Florida Regional Medical Program to get organized than it had its counterpart in Georgia. Florida received its first planning grant on November 1, 1967, beginning operations March 1, 1969. [22]

Dr. Clyde M. Collins, editor of the Journal of the Florida Medical Association, stated some of the reasons for Florida's problem. Some of them stemmed from the "vagueness of the legislation as it was written and to the differences of opinion of people interpreting the law as to how to accomplish its objectives." [23] Otherwise, "beset by the lack of understanding on the part of the private practitioner, false accusations from the lay press, the aggressiveness of our medical schools in obtaining their share of available largesse, personality conflicts among full-time and volunteer members, and a paucity of tangible results, the Florida Regional Medical Program is entering its third year" -- apparently in his view without much to show for it. [24]

Things seemed to be getting out of hand in Dr. Collins's view: "Grant funds, provided for planning and operational phases, were not intended to be a method of paying medical care nor designed specifically to build hospitals, laboratories and medical schools but to preserve the traditional relationship between the patient and his physician... No one is against improving health services, but is this the best way to do it?" [25] Dr. Collins seemed to be working himself up. He continued: "The history of our nation is filled with the cadaverous remains of federal bureaucracies based on idealistic methods of serving urgent social problems which failed as expensive boondoggles because in practice the solution to the local parts of the problem did not fit into the federally proposed molds." [26]

In the planning phase, the Florida RMP divided itself into three regions: South Florida, centered at the University of Miami Medical School; Mid-Florida, centered at the medical school at University of South Florida at Tampa; and North Florida, headquartered in the Medical School of the University of Florida at Gainesville. By 1970, a subregional pattern was agreed to which gave greater emphasis to what the Journal of the Florida Medical Association termed "community involvement." Seven district offices were established; Pensacola, Tallahassee, Jacksonville, Daytona Beach, Orlando, Tampa, Fort Meyers, West Palm Beach, Miami-Broward County, and Miami-Monroe County. The Medical Association didn't want to crow about breaking the grip of the medical schools but the Journal did note with approval that the new arrangement would bring continuing education down to the local level, bolster community hospitals, and permit local assumption of responsibility of developing operational projects. [27]

As in other places, the early emphasis was on heart disease, cancer, stroke, kidney disease, with a diabetes emphasis added later. With respect to coronary care, a variety of programs were undertaken, including what was thought to be a very important training of coronary care nurses. However, the effort met with some disappointment due to "recruiting difficulties and unwillingness of hospital administrators to allow nurses a leave of absence for four weeks of training." [28] This was true even though RMP funds would pay half the cost of such training with the other half being paid by the hospital or some other community resources. Nonetheless, some 500 CCU nurses were trained in three years. [29]

Eventually, the Florida Program gained cohesion, and individual physicians, not necessarily reflecting the view of the Florida Medical Association, came on board. For example, some 500 Floridians gradually participated in the program as advisors, either to the state, regional or district programs. Looking on the bright side, the Chairman and Deputy Director of the Florida Regional Medical Program argued that the RMP concept "is almost tailor-made for Florida." [30] State law had banned the dissection of the human body until the 1950's. This effectively discouraged the establishment of a medical school in the state, and left Florida far behind its southeastern neighbors not only in medical research and education but in tertiary level care resources as well. [31]

The Florida Program made special note of the recent and rapid advances, many originating in and from the National Institutes of Health in the treatment of cancer and children, in both leukemias and solid tumors. Hence, it funded several centers around the State to which physicians could refer patients whom they suspected of having cancer for confirmation of diagnosis, and for development of multiple treatment modes and schedules which could then be administered by the child's physician. Such referring consultation services were set up in Tampa, Miami, Jacksonville and Gainesville. Other programs included those in neo-natal care. Here also was a case in which "Florida's past record... can scarcely be viewed with pride." In 1970, Flordia ranked 39th among all states in infant mortality. After the establishment of the new RMP program in neo-natal care, the number of neo-natal deaths dropped from a four year period from 1,848 in 1970 to 1,389 in 1974. [32]

Another unusual program, in the array of medical programs sponsored by RMPs across the country including Florida, was focused on hospital- acquired infections, a problem not considered by the President's Commission on Heart Disease, Cancer and Stroke, but which, in that period, was causing some 50,000 deaths a year in the U.S., roughly the same number of deaths as from automobile accidents. [33]

The most impressive of Florida's programs was development of the State's first emergency medical services. It took four years to get it organized, but the medical statistic that drove its establishment remained static and frightening: "25,000 of the 40,000 deaths from heart disease occurred within the first hour after the onset of symptoms." [34] In 1970, this prompted a major investment by RMP in this area. In consultation with the Florida Medical Association, the State Division of Health, the Florida Hospital Association, the medical schools and others, the plan was completed with RMP funds and presented to the Governor and the legislature which adopted it and funded it. As in other parts of the Country, the EMS system in Florida proved successful in significantly reducing the number of such deaths.

These achievements and others gradually gained the approval of the health care establishment, finally including the Florida Medical Association, for the Florida Regional Medical Program. Still, the program continued to feel the heat from a variety of sources. One area in which leadership continued to feel defensive was in operational costs. In a report in 1975, the leaders asserted: "From the beginning, it's been a cardinal rule of FRMP's operation to keep its staff small, but highly skilled, and to keep its operating overhead at the lowest possible level... RMP has also endeavored to cooperate fully with physicians and other health professional groups and institutions and to avoid duplication and overlap of existing facilities and services...." [35] But in Florida, as elsewhere among state programs, and consequently nationally, the overhead cost somehow represented a vulnerable point.

The Florida Medical Association mellowed a bit over time. The subsequent editor of its journal, Dr. J. Franz Stewart of Coral Gables, seemed more favorable to RMP than his predecessor Dr. Collins. Dr. Collins was still shaking his head in 1971 about the meaning and effectiveness of the program: "In spite of confusion over goals of the program itself and in spite of not having reached the average practitioner, yet not condoning the high administrative costs and seeing no valid arguments on any conflicts of interest, in a meeting last month, the Board of Directors of FRMP reaffirmed their belief in the program and their confidence in its officers." [36]

In Florida, from beginning to end, the emphasis -- almost as if it were put in boldface cap -- was on "assisting physicians" and others in their delivery of care. In Georgia, using this same formulation, the emphasis in a parallel phrase seemed to be on "enhancing care for people."

Notes:

1. J. Gordon Barrow, "Georgia Regional Medical Program - Off and Running," Journal of the Medical Association of Aug. 1967. See also: Barrow article on Georgia RMP, in Special Edition on Regional Medical Programs in Postgraduate Medicine, 1967; Louis L Bettey, "Georgia Regional Medical Program," Journal of Medical Association of Georgia, April 1967.
2. Interview with Dr. Barrow, March 16, 1992.
3. Ibid.
4. Innovative Plans for the Georgia Regional Medical Programs," Excerpts from GRMP Program Grant Applications, Journal of the Medical Association of Georgia, April 1967, p. 149.
5. Ibid.
6. Ibid., p. 150.
7. Interview with Dr. Barrow.
8. "Innovative Plans," op. cit., p. 150.

9. Ibid.

10. Barrow, "Georgia Medical Program - Off and Running," op. cit., p. 337.

11. "Innovative Plans," op. cit., p. 149.

12. Interview with Dr. Barrow

13. J. Gordon Barrow, "Health Access Stations," Journal of the Medical Association of Georgia, Feb. 1973.

14. Ibid., p. 48.

15. Ibid.

16. Ibid., p.49.

17. Interview with Dr. Barrow.

18. Ibid.

19. Ibid.

20. Journal of the Medical Association of Georgia, June 1976, Vol. 65, p. 193.

21. "Medical school Professor Recognized," EmoKy Alumnus, October 1976.

22. U.S. DHEW, Division of Regional Medical Programs, Director of Regional Medical Programs, 1969.

23. "F.R.M.P.," editorial, Journal of the Florida Medical Association, Feb. 1971, p. 44.

24. Ibid.

25. Ibid.

26. Ibid.

27. Granville W. Larrimore, G.R. Eugebretson, and C.E. Moore, "Florida Regional Medical Program - An Overview," Journal of the Florida Medical Association, May 1973.

28. F.R.M.P., editorial, opt. cit., pg 46

29. G.R. Eugebretson, Granville W. Larrimore, and Coyle Moore, "The Florida Regional Medical Program: A Report," Journal of the Florida Medical Association, Dec. 1975, p. 45.

30. Ibid.

31. Ibid.

32. Ibid.

33. Ibid., p. 46.

34. Ibid., p. 47.

35. Ibid.

36. Editorial, Journal of the Florida Medical Association, Feb. 1971.

Chapter 8

Alabama

Alabama was among those few states that had a dual, very important advantage: the Regional Medical Program was contiguous with state boundaries, and within the state there was a single medical school. In the case of the University of Alabama School of Medicine, most doctors practicing in the state were its alumni.

An additional political advantage was the unique situation in Alabama where the State Board of Health was comprised of the entire membership of the Medical Association of the State of Alabama (MASA). Between annual meetings the Board of Censors of MASA served as the State Committee on Public Health (with no non-physician members!) and also as the Board of Medical Examiners. Thus the Health Department and the Medical Association spoke with one voice, unlike most other states.

There was also an historical advantage in political terms. The senior U.S. senator from Alabama, Lister Hill, was one of the leading proponents of a strong federal role in health. Beginning with his partnership with Senator Harold Burton of Ohio in proposing the Hill-Burton Hospital Construction Act of 1946, and continuing through his years as principal Senate proponent of the National Institutes of Health, his colleagues in the Senate had referred to him as "Mr. Health." Given his interests, Hill had the great advantage of serving as chair of both the Committee on Labor and Welfare and of the Health subcommittee of the Appropriations Committee. The Senator kept in constant communication with health leaders in the state, particularly in the medical school. There had to have been a predisposition, in that important circle, to embrace the new federal program.[1]

A particular part of the general political advantage was that the president of the University of Alabama Birmingham, Dr. Joseph Volker, Dean of the School of Dentistry before assuming the top post at the University, and Dr. S. Richardson Hill, Dean of the Medical School, subsequently Vice President for Health Affairs and later President of UAB, had long served in advisory posts at the federal level. More than many medical academicians, they kept close track of new federal health initiatives. Their aptitude in doing so, and their persuasive powers even with the generally conservative state legislature, made the University of Alabama School of Medicine an increasingly important institution in the state and region, and a beacon for very distinguished surgeons, physicians, and health care administrators from all over the country.[2]

One of the latter who had recently come to Birmingham and the medical center was Dr. Benjamin Wells, who for many years had been one of the senior administrators of the Veterans Administration Medical System, that extensive system of hospitals which, by the 1960's, were affiliated with medical schools across the country. These three men, President Volker, Vice President Hill, and Dr. Wells were the planners of the Alabama RMP. They brought in others from the University and around the state.[3]

The first decision was to make Ben Wells the Director of the Alabama Regional Medical Programs. His first decision was to recruit the out-going president of the Medical Association of the State of Alabama, Dr. J. L.. Finney, as Deputy Director. Together the two men involved the heads of the statewide Heart Association and Cancer Society, and the State of Alabama Health Department. They also involved a few business men whose qualifications included -- but definitely were not limited to -- their own networks in the corporate and civic sectors and all of who were big Alabama boosters. (One of these, Winton Blount, would become Postmaster General in the next national administration, that of Richard Nixon.) Not only was the state medical society supportive of the new program, but as the second and long-time director of the Alabama Regional Medical Program, Dr. John Packard, later put it: The practicing physicians across the state were "too few and too busy to be defensive." Instead they were "grateful for any help" anybody would give them.[4]

With respect to the paucity of physicians, of Alabama's 67 counties, one had no physician, several had only two or three, and another twenty or so had but a few. The concentrations of the practicing physicians were in the larger cities -- Birmingham, Montgomery, Mobile, Huntsville -- and the problem of geographical distribution was as keen or keener than anywhere in the country.

The political sophisticates organizing the program knew that the challenge of doing so would not be enormous. But they also knew exactly what must be done and they proceeded to do it sure-footedly and ultimately successfully. Beyond including all the major figures in the health care, health policy and health administration areas, from an early point they focused on priorities and approaches that emphasized the obvious: heart disease, cancer and stroke. They knew that health care personnel other than physicians were essential, especially in a state with an underpopulation of doctors.

They also knew that there was not big money to be had through Regional Medical Programs. They knew this in several ways, first because the medical school faculty was, even in the 1960's, receiving very significant support through research grants from the National Institutes of Health. Further, the school itself was receiving a fair amount in health manpower training. Thus the one or two million dollars a year which might come to the Alabama Regional Medical Program was never seen as financially central to the medical school's future. Indeed, the Alabama RMP leaders' recognition of the fiscal reality and the articulation of that reality to everyone who got involved -- from medical school faculty to community hospitals applying for grants -- helped to ensure that few if any unrealistic expectations were generated.[5]

Beginning in 1968 and continuing through 1972, the total funds awarded to the Alabama Regional Medical Program, and most of it in turn to projects, totaled just over $3 million. This sum, Dr. Packard later specified, amounted to "almost exactly twenty cents per citizen per year."[6] Inasmuch as this relatively modest funding had been anticipated, it compelled RMP to give to potential applicants two "directions" simultaneously. The first was to advise virtually every group applying for project funds to submit the leanest possible budget -- and not even think about spending large sums of money for new equipment! Second, if the budget was out of line with guidelines, the rest of the funds would have to come from other sources. The other pattern which recognition of fiscal realities encouraged was that of supporting complementary efforts. For example, the ARMP joined with the Appalachian Regional Commission in a program to encourage physicians to locate in rural counties of the northwestern part of the state.

Despite the controversy that arose when the original legislation was introduced in Congress, regarding whether the program would affect traditional patterns of medical care and the consequent prohibition on the activities that might do so, the Alabama regional advisory group set certain objectives and arranged them in priority order. "These objectives are: 1) improvement of the delivery of health care especially emergency medical care and care in rural areas; 2) manpower development; and 3) continuing education."[7]

The concrete programs undertaken in pursuit of these aims included one simple one which had an unusual twist. While the first emphasis was on the killer diseases, there was an underlying need: Not since the public health surveys of the Depression years had there been a systematic county-by-county assessment of medical resources and health care needs of the people of the state. Thus one of the first projects developed and funded by ARMP was such a survey. To do so, the program had enlisted an important, established, well-respected and completely non-threatening network of professionals, the county agricultural agents. If not unique, this was most unusual and in a quiet way, most inventive. As Dr. Packard said many times, the whole approach of the Alabama RMP was to be helpful but not threatening.

Another obvious need in Alabama as elsewhere was for emergency medical services. This situation also reflected the dispersal of population, sometimes in communities far from a well-equipped hospitals or even community hospitals with emergency care capacity. Regarding training, the program helped develop and sponsor the training of allied health personnel that linked UAB's Regional Technical Institute with the 18 junior colleges in the state.

Early in the ARMP's tenure, a model system was developed with its support by the Birmingham Emergency Medical Services Committee, with equal attention given to emergency medical training for technicians and to transportation of the critically ill. Professional EMS team members from the system actually went on the road to do demonstrations in cities throughout the state, often resulting in the formation of local EMS Committees made up of professionals from existing hospitals or clinics and fire and police departments. This activity actually spurred the development of legislation which, enacted in 1971, required licensure of ambulance services and the establishment of a State Emergency Medical Services Advisory Board to function under the State Board of Health. Rules, regulations and standards were in effect by 1973 and helped direct subsequent ARMP projects as to transportation, communication and EMS training.[8]

Projects concerning the care and transportation of the critically ill newborns were a prominent part of the EMS Services. They addressed the particular needs of these tiny patients through the establishment of levels of care nurseries in cities of Alabama, education of nurses and physicians for these nurseries and transportation of the babies to the appropriate nursery.

Among other simple but imaginative programs which began fairly early was the Medical Information Service via Telephone (MIST). This too related to the origins of the national program, and specifically the information gap perceived by President Johnson between the best most advanced knowledge at the fingertips of the most advanced scientists and practitioners on the one hand, and on the other, the understanding and capacity of physicians far removed from centers of medical excellence. The Alabama telephone service was the brain child of Dr. Cliff Meador, Dean of the medical school, and it was overseen, expanded and refined over the next decade by Dr. Margaret S. Klapper of the medical faculty who was to become, in 1973, Executive Director of ARMP. It involved, on the one side, primarily internists, cardiologists, oncologists and pediatric physicians on the medical school faculty; on the other side were physicians serving in small towns and rural areas. As it was subsequently described:

"The operation of this program is relatively simple. Incoming and outgoing Watts lines with accompanying syntrex tie lines and a recorder comprised the hardware. An administrative assistant from the division of continuing education coordinates the endeavor. And an operator sufficiently knowledgeable in the medical sciences to "field" the calls and pick out the personnel. This operator is on duty from 8am to 5pm five days a week.... Faculty participate through a structured on-call scheduling and electronic alerting devices help assure promptness of response. The pilot study program included at first four counties, one rural, one urban, and two intermediate-sized.[9]

In the beginning phase, there were various concerns about the efficacy of the program. Would the whole plan be viewed simply as a scheme to increase referrals to the medical center? Would practicing specialists consider their consultative fees in jeopardy? Would enthusiasm of the program wane? Would persons other than practitioners and health professionals learn the telephone number, seek information and use it unethically or otherwise adversely? Would practitioners object to identifying themselves and object to having their advice recorded? The recording was included as part of the program, so that excerpts could be analyzed for modifications of the program and for educational planning.

Toward the end of the six-month pilot period, it was clear that physicians from all over the state were participating. Within the first two years, almost 35% of the practicing physicians in the state outside of Birmingham (who would not need to use a Watts line) had used the system. More than 100 faculty members had responded to more than 1200 calls, and more that three thousand pages of library material had been sent as follow up to the telephone consultations.

Gradually MIST was extended. As Dr. Klapper recalls: "It lent itself well to other feasibility studies such as MIST-VAH (linking the VA hospitals to the medical center) and MIST-TRI, attempting EKG transmission via telephone from 3 counties. MIST facilitated what we referred to as shared patient care whereby the patient could be cared for by the local physician with periodic visits to the medical center; the local physician and faculty physician communicated via MIST."[10] MIST was very quickly made available to all health professionals. The tape libraries for physicians and nurses were purchased through the Wisconsin RMP and utilized until Wisconsin discontinued it. Monitoring of MIST calls very quickly went from recording to data sheets and punch cards, to computer record keeping.

When ARMP terminated in 1976, 130,575 MIST calls had been processed. But the program continued in Alabama and, with support from the National Institutes of Health and its National Library of Medicine, expanded elsewhere.

Within a few years, MIST ceased to depend upon the hospital operators to handle night and week-end calls and the MIST operation became available "around-the-clock". It housed the Dial Access Tapes Library of the Southern Medical Association for a number of years. It remains the access line for the critical-care Transport Services of the University of Alabama Medical Center, with its national reach. MIST celebrated its thirtieth anniversary in 1999.

The physician shortage in Alabama also meant that the emphasis on training programs for nurses, physicians' assistants, and other allied health personnel was embraced by physicians. In Alabama as in many other places, the Regional Medical Program established a consistent pattern and advantage in the first five years. By supporting dialogues, planning sessions, and overall communication between and among professional groups not accustomed to such on a regular basis, but seeming to welcome it, it brought the University and its medical school closer to professional people all over the state.

The interaction went further. Before the end of the program, not only was ARMP participating in regular planning activities with the State Board of Health, but also with the Comprehensive Health Planning agency. All the federally supported health program administrators met together from time to time. As Dr. Packard remarked: "We were in bed together as well as working in the field together."[11] What he may have had specifically in mind was that the nurse educator in charge of personnel training programs for the Regional Medical Program was married to a physician who directed the State C.H.P. But beyond that, communication and cooperation between the Alabama Regional Medical Program and all the other agencies concerned with health matters remained remarkably consistent and constructive from beginning to end.

One of the most unusual collaborations was that involving the county agents, who had been recruited to undertake the early health needs survey. Called the Health Extension Learning Program (HELP), this was a cooperative effort of Aurburn University Extension Division, the State Board of Health and the School of Community and Allied Health Resources (now the School of Related Health Sciences) at UAB, beginning in 1971. The Dean of the School of Medicine, Dr. Meador -- the son of a veterinarian also worked with the Agricultural Extension Service -- conceived the idea, and all parties agreed to try it.

Dr. Margaret Klapper summarized this idea: "This network of county agents had completely eradicated hog cholera from Alabama by including education of the rural public as the only added ingredient [to the scientific effort]. Why then should a state of affairs be tolerated wherein the farmers knew more about the health of their livestock than about their children, themselves and their families? Project HELP operated upon the premise that the approach to human disease does not differ fundamentally from that successfully used in animal husbandry." [12]

Topics addressed through HELP included emergency and acute care; preventative dental practices; arthritis awareness; cancer awareness and early detection. The mechanism which operated in project HELP provided a stable vehicle through which almost any health education or disease prevention program could be implemented.

Before the Alabama RMP was forced to cease operations in October 1976, it had, during nine active years, funded over 100 programs. A number of them were continued with other support, often that of the University of Alabama at Birmingham. Some, such as the MIST program and several Area Health Education Programs, continue today.

Notes:

An adaptation of this chapter was published in the Winter 1995-96 issue of "Alabama Medicine," The Journal of the Medical Association of Alabama.

1. As a native Alabaman sometimes assisting in the political representations of Alabama in Washington, the author followed closely the development of the University of Alabama in Birmingham and especially its school of Medicine. In those years (1959-65), and subsequently as a scholar, the author chronicled the health-related accomplishments of Senator Lister Hill, in part in a book on which was returned to as a resource for relevant situations, including this chapter. See Stephen P. Strickland, *Politics, Science and Dread Disease* (Cambridge: Harvard University Press), 1972.
2. Interviews with Dr. Hill in 1992 and 1993. On file in RMP Archives of Regional Medical Programs, National Library of Medicine.
3. Ibid.
4. Interview with Dr. John Packard, April 1992. See also interview with Dr. Packard conducted bye Dr. Donald A.B. Lindberg, November 1991, RMP Archives of NLM.
5. Interviews with Dr. Hill and Dr. Packard.

76

6. John M. Packard, M.D., "What Is the Alabama Regional Medical Program and Its Practical Application to Rural Health?" Journal of the Medical Association of Alabama, December 1972, p.427.

7. Ibid., p. 430.

8. Information provided in correspondence (and related materials) with author Margaret S. Klapper, M.D.., member of the faculty and Assistant Vice President for Health Affairs of the University of Alabama School of Medicine, Dr. Klapper served as directory of ARMP from 1973 to 1976 when it ceased operations.

9. William F. Bridgers, M.D., et. al, "Project Help," University of Alabama in Birmingham, Alabama file, RMP Archives, NLM.

10. Correspondence with Dr. Klapper. See also Margaret S. Klapper, M.D., "Medical Information Service via Telephone (MIST),'- Journal of the Medical Association of the State of Alabama. October 1970, pp. 257-269.

11. Correspondence with Dr. Klapper.

12. Correspondence with Dr. Klapper.

Chapter 9

Missouri

Dean Vernon Wilson of the University of Missouri School of Medicine learned of the imminent adoption of the Heart Disease, Cancer and Stroke amendments at a meeting of the Association of American Medical Schools Executive Council on February 6, 1965. Dr. William Stewart, HEW staff man for the legislation initiative and soon to be the Surgeon General of the Public Health Service, had come to tell the medical school deans about the legislation. He asked them to testify in favor of it when Senator Hill held hearings -- the very next week.

Vern Wilson had one concern. Since arriving in Columbia from Kansas to become Dean a few years before, he had been making a strenuous effort to build links between the School of Medicine and the practicing physicians of the state. He did so by getting in his single-engine plane and flying off "to meet with every county medical society that would have him."[1] This in itself impressed the doctors of Missouri. One recollection is of a group of doctors, after one meeting, driving Dr. Wilson to Dr. Billy Jack Bass' private airstrip in Salem and turning their cars at right angles towards a make-shift runway so as to illuminate his departure with their headlights.

Dr. Wilson formed an advisory council made up of the medical society presidents. His efforts seemed to be working. He and his staff colleagues were building a statewide network to deal with Missouri's health problems. So he wanted to be sure the new program he heard Bill Stewart describing in Washington didn't mean that he would have to start over, following a detailed and elaborate new set of federal rules and procedures as to how to build a regional medical program. Not at all, Dr.

Stewart responded. The idea was to embrace and build on existing cooperative networks whenever possible.[2]   Thus reassured and accepting the word of Bill Stewart that the bill would quickly become law, Dean Wilson returned to Columbia, gathered his colleagues together, and began planning with renewed vigor.

Those on whom Dr. Wilson had already been relying and who now joined the newly focused enterprise recall their early conversations with Dr. Wilson as having occurred before anyone else in the State -- doctors, congressmen, newspaper reporters, lobbyists -- evidenced any awareness of yet another Great Society Health proposal shaping up. Perhaps this is not so surprising, given that only one month had elapsed between the time of the DeBakey Commission report to the President and the submission of legislation to implement it. Further, the attention-grabbing controversy initiated by the American Medical Association had not yet erupted.

Dr. Wilson had only been in Missouri a few years, but he seemed to know the state like the palm of his hand. Forming a team to do a job seemed to have been second nature to him. And though he later denied any awareness of political considerations, he was by all accounts a master strategist and a powerful persuader. One has the image of him as an imaginative but selective, modest but compelling pied piper, playing his tune to one listener, or one small audience, at a time. It was a very different style from LBJ's, but it had the same effect: Almost all who heard his plea succumbed.[3]

Within a few weeks, Wilson had gotten journalists, engineers, computer experts, public relations professionals, nurses and public officials to join medical doctors and osteopathic physicians (the latter combination being in itself an almost miraculous union) to "think positive" about what a Missouri Regional Medical Program could do for the state, its people and its institutions of higher learning.

One of Dr. Wilson's first recruits was Bill Allen (Dr. William C.) who until 1965 served with the State Health Department while also a member of the clinical faculty at the University of Missouri Medical School. In that job he had come to be acquainted with many physicians throughout the state as well as all of the hospital and nursing home administrators and those who ran and sat on the boards of the professional health associations such as the Cancer Society and the Heart Association.

By the time President Johnson's signature was dry on P.L. 89-239, Dr. Allen was installed in the Dean's office, collecting every piece of information he could about the DeBakey Commission, the legislative history, and the views of affected professionals concerning the Heart, Cancer and Stroke Act of 1965.

Fortunately, he says, the advisory committee to the Dean of the School of Medicine not only had on it the county medical society presidents but all living ex-presidents of the Missouri Medical Association. And it was soon to have other key figures in the medical community, including Mrs. Harry Truman's personal physician. When the law passed, Dr. Allen recalled: "We called the group together and told them about the Heart, Cancer and Stroke legislation and that it appeared it would soon be funded. We asked them to decide whether we should be involved and how we should go about it. So the Medical Advisory Committee said they indeed wanted to give it a try."[4]

Dean Wilson found another advantage. The University acquired a couple of DC-3s. He dispatched teams to Chicago, the Mayo Clinic and other points East to look at some reputedly interesting innovations in patient care delivery being undertaken at several hospitals. He and Dr. Allen took another trip to St. Louis to visit the medical school deans at Washington and St. Louis universities. Missouri ought to have a statewide program, they thought, and they knew that the participation of the other medical schools was essential. Washington U.'s Dean Kenton King and St. Louis' Bob Felix -- earlier the first director of the National Institute of Mental Health -- both responded positively. But both said they would "have to run this by" their faculties.

"Running by" turned out to involve "flying back," with the Columbia initiators returning to St. Louis to talk directly with the medical faculty department heads. Dr. Allen suggests that there was no special resistance to the concept or the substance of the program, but there was one question and answer that thwarted their hopes. The chairmen asked: "Are you going to be involved with the various medical societies?" Dr. Wilson answered: "We will not go one foot without the full cooperation of the medical societies." The chairmen said: "Then we want no part of your program."[5] St. Louis would organize its own regional medical program, serving its traditional constituency in the metropolitan area, including Illinois counties across the Mississippi. Still, there developed regular communication and frequent cooperation between the two programs.

Kansas City would also be a bit difficult. The city straddled a state line and, in Kansas, a regional medical program was also getting underway under the leadership of Dr. Charles Lewis, at the University of Kansas Medical Center. And under the University of Missouri system, on the Missouri side of the line, plans had been laid to build a new and different kind of medical school, a two-year program extending from the basic university curriculum and integrated with it. This concept was novel, and those leading its development had an array of obstacles to overcome, as everybody in the Kansas city area and throughout the state knew. Whether they would lend their weight to a new state-wide program centered in the medical school in Columbia was a serious question. But Dr. Wilson and his colleagues were persuasive. They gave assurances that they would work cooperatively with Kansas RMP, and that the Missouri RMP would give special attention to the needs of the new medical education and training enterprise in Kansas City.

Simultaneously with the visits to his fellow medical school deans, Dr. Wilson and his colleagues talked with medical society chairmen, in group as the advisory council to the dean and, in many cases, individually as well. All agreed on the value of a state-wide approach. In fact, the dean's advisory council made up as powerful a state-wide network as could be assembled. Consulting with the council meant reaching into every medical community and region in the state.

With wide support thus garnered, the Missouri Regional Medical Program could go forward. The center of planning and strategy was Columbia, but from the very first, ideas for it, including proposals for medical delivery innovations, came from all over the state. There would be programs in every part of the state: Springfield, Kirksville, the Ozark Region, the Bootheel Region, Hannibal, Cape Girardeau, Skaggs, Lakes County, Dunklin County, the Green Hills area in the North Central part of the state, Cedar County, Callaway.

In addition to the medical societies and medical leaders of the various geographical regions, the Columbia team also enlisted from the very beginning the leadership of the health associations, including the Missouri Hospital Association, the Statewide Heart Association, the Cancer Society, and the Kidney Foundation. Dr. George Wakerlin, the first director of the Missouri program, reported that beyond the Advisory Council, the program had established a Scientific Review Committee (which included among others all the medical school deans and representative of the state health agencies) and a Liaison Committee which was composed of representatives of 20 state organizations in the health field including professional societies.[6]

These organizations were enlisted not only for their ideas and political strength throughout the state, but in order that, from an early point, they might run programs in their medical and organizational areas of expertise. Over the eight active grant-making years of the Missouri Regional Medical Program, the Missouri Heart Association, the Kidney Foundation, the Missouri State Medical Association, the Missouri Nursing Home Association, as well as an assortment of general and specialized colleges and schools, organized and ran programs under the aegis of, and with funding through, the Missouri RMP.

The organization of headquarters was equally interesting, perhaps more so. Naturally, Dr. Wilson asked his medical colleagues to join in the effort and enlisted associates in the Schools of Nursing and of Allied Health. But he reached beyond the traditional collaborators and sought out those with professional expertise in what were, at that moment in history, fields utterly unrelated to the improvement of health care and the development of medical programs for people. Among early recruits for the team was Bill Kimel, Dean of the College of Engineering; and department chairs in engineering including Cyrus Harbourt from Electrical and Computer Engineering, Jay Goldman from Industrial Engineering, and Gayle Adams, Director of the Engineering Computer Center.

Dean Kimel remembers Dr. Wilson especially encouraging him and Dean William Moyer of the School of Medicine, both appointed as deans in 1968, to work together and to get their respective faculties to do so. The cooperation was remarkable and productive, and engendered particular teamwork efforts -- such as that between Dr. Donald Lindberg and Dr. Samuel J. Dwyer, Director of Bioengineering, in developing computer applications to medical science.

The University of Missouri is nationally famous for its school of journalism; so its dean, Dr. Will Stevenson, and key faculty were asked to join in shaping the new program. Vernon Wilson knew that systematic communication with various professional and political power centers and with the public was essential. Not forgetting the simpler traditions of communication, Dr. Wilson recruited a public information officer Fred Frazier, whose career had been in public relations.

There was obviously extraordinary talent within the University and within the state, but Dr. Wilson had a long reach as well as a good eye for talent. In addition to Dr. Wakerlin and others with particular specialties, Dr. Wilson also recruited Dr. Arthur E. Rikli, who had worked in regional medical networks for some years as the regional consultant in chronic disease for the Public Health Service and subsequently as chief of the National Heart Disease control program, based in the Washington headquarters of the PHS. Dr. Rikli had also worked on the computerization of electrocardiograms. He had had experience with the Hill-Burton program and truly knew the country as whole. When Dr. George Wakerlin became Director, Dr. Rikli become Coordinator.

Twenty-five years after the close of the RMP, all the Missourians give Buck Rikli great credit for helping insure that what Dr. Wilson, Dr. Allen, Dr. Lindberg and the other remarkable initial team had started continued to run smoothly and consistently and successfully for the next decade. Dr. Rikli continued to carry on regional activities begun under the Missouri RMP, in 1975 becoming coordinator of the Missouri Kidney Program and otherwise remaining involved in health care in the state.

The enterprise authorized by The Heart Disease, Cancer and Stroke Act of 1965 officially only took a few months to organize. The national plan was officially in place -- despite lots of scurrying and almost continual modifications -- by 1966. One of the first regional programs to receive a planning grant was Missouri, on July 1 of that year. By April 1967, the Missouri Regional Program began making grants, putting it ahead of most other regional medical programs in the country by a year.[7]

As has been illustrated, a few others also got off to a strong and rapid start. But the great majority of RMPs did not get organized nearly as early, and even if they did, were not in a position to make grants and start programs until the middle of 1968. Whether its quick start helped Missouri become one of the best recognized Regional Medical Programs in the country is not absolutely certain, but compared to the histories of other programs, the swift, comprehensive and meticulous consultation and planning that took place were extraordinary.

When he had consolidated the support of the professional constituencies and a state-wide community base, Dr. Wilson went to the Governor, then Warren Hearns, and asked him to appoint members the Regional Advisory Group (RAG) to the Missouri Regional Medical Program. The governor agreed, and selected as chairman Nathan Stark. The governor further agreed to appoint one of three names proposed for each spot on the RAG by Dr. Wilson and his colleagues. The Missouri program was deemed to be so promising that another exceptional phenomenon subsequently occurred: The state legislator who represented Northeast Columbia, Representative Harold Volkmer, went to work to get himself appointed to the Advisory Committee, apparently wanting to be a part of a winning as well as a pioneering enterprise.[8] Later Mr. Volkmer was elected to Congress, representing the 9th District of Missouri.

One of the original impulses behind RMP was probably related to Lyndon Johnson's heart attack. The President's excellent and swift recovery, he properly recognized, was due to excellent and immediate medical attention and treatment. In those years, thirty-five years ago, heart attacks were frequently accompanied by death. This was because medical attention was not always swift, particularly outside urban areas where transportation to hospitals was not fast, and because treatment modes were not advanced. The President whose best policies grew out of his own personal experiences — whether in education, the treatment of minorities, or health care -- did not want any American suffering a heart attack to die simply because the person could not reach the hospital, or doctors could not reach the person, quickly enough.

However the programmatic emphases of RMP might expand and shift over the next few years, the Missouri RMP leaders obviously recognized the central purpose. From the beginning, Missouri RMP spent funds trying to help the President achieve one of his first objectives. Early on, joined by the State Health department, Missouri RMP surveyed the approximately 186 hospitals in the state to determine how many of them had intensive care units or at least an intensive care capability. Out of that number, only 15 had such units or capability in 1966. An obvious question was why, when intensive care units had already shown in other places how effective they could be in restoring desperately ill patients to normalcy, Missouri hospitals had not proceeded to create them. The typical reply was two-fold: not enough money and no trained personnel.

One of the early Missouri RMP programs was to set up an intensive care unit to serve as a model for the rest of the state. It included a training program at the University hospital in Columbia, to which all the other hospitals were invited to select and send appropriate personnel from their staffs, and to pay for that training. Dr. Bill Allen recalls: "They spent two weeks at the model program here in Columbia and then would go back and spend a month at their own hospitals, do correspondence courses in that period of time, work to develop intensive care units in their hospitals, and then come back to Columbia for a final two weeks of advanced training."[9] (Those trained in intensive care included a lot of nurses as well as physicians). The other essential components were: properly equipped ambulances -- provided by hospitals rather than by morticians which up to then was typical Missouri practice; and expanded CPR training so that those first reaching heart attack and other victims would know how to respond. It took other resources to achieve the overall objective, but in the next decade, practically all the hospitals had developed an intensive care capability.

Another problem in medical treatment in the 1960's was, as President Johnson also noted pointedly, the extraordinary range of new medical knowledge being developed. Much of it emanated from the National Institutes of Health, in its laboratories and or with its support at the principal medical school centers across the country. The centers did not often have ways of sharing these advances with primary care physicians in most American communities. Despite some defensive professional views about the matter, there was significant agreement that even the best trained and greatly skilled physicians could have a difficult time keeping up with new advances, if they were not themselves attached to the principal medical complexes of their regions. As Dr. Wilson put it: "Any physician trying to carry around in his head all of the knowledge that is needed for even a single medical discipline is just destined for an end."[10] Various approaches to this problem were developed. In Missouri (as in Alabama, Wisconsin and elsewhere) one of them was a simple matter of installing a telephone link between every community in the state with groups of specialists in Columbia, Kansas City or St. Louis.

Another novelty of the Missouri RMP – which became a major effort -- was the development and use of computers. Dr. Wilson had a strong hunch that communications with respect to medical problems and solutions could be facilitated and expanded through the use of computers. In this connection, one of the first physicians in his own school he talked to was a young pathologist who had already begun using computers as an aid to the categorization and diagnosis of diseases. That person was Dr. Donald A. B. Lindberg. In one of his last commentaries on Regional Medical Programs, an interview with Dr. Lindberg in 1991, Dr. Wilson said "My initial impression of RMP was that it could be a tool that would help us take technical knowledge and make it work in the health care system."[11] In Missouri, it did.

From his side, when Don Lindberg was invited to join the University of Missouri School of Medicine Pathology Department in 1960, one of the early conversations that intrigued him was with the Dean-designate of the school, Vernon Wilson. Dr. Lindberg had already been impressed with the opportunity the department chairman had offered, namely that he could continue to carry out his biological research and also run the clinical pathology laboratory for the University Hospital. But he and Dr. Wilson talked about the need for putting electronic communications systems, still in their infancy, to work to serve medical needs.[12]

Earlier that year, Dr. Lindberg had been on the site visit team for the National Institutes of Health, looking at a potential grant to Massachusetts General Hospital and its medical director, Dr. John Knowles, for exploring possibilities of the use of computers in medicine. That early work had gone on relatively well, if in very rudimentary ways. But the real question, in those days, was whether there was any market for using computer systems in medicine. Dr. Lindberg was impressed that Dr. Wilson, himself trained in pharmacology, thought the answer was definitely a yes. This was unusual, because outside of "Mass General," nobody in medicine seemed remotely interested in the matter.

Missouri proved a challenging place. But for a young man with a wide range of interests and enormous energy, it also proved to be frustrating. Running two labs was somewhat tougher than Dr. Lindberg had imagined, especially since he felt so keenly the dual obligation involved, one to his NIH supporters and one to the patients. The diagnosis of those patients' conditions and the analysis of what treatment might work was at least a matter of sickness or health, if not of life or death. Related to all of this was a philosophical conviction about medicine, and how the University of Missouri Hospital approached medical care. That approach was that the hospital ought to be able to provide every person that came into it with excellent care across the board. Other hospitals, including notable ones in the East where Dr. Lindberg had served, in fact had the capacity to provide the very best care in the world. And they did so for anyone who could pay for it. But Missouri had good specialists, good facilities and, in those days, even before Medicare and Medicaid reimbursements, the inclination to take care of its patients in a comprehensive way.

The dual laboratory burden accelerated Dr. Lindberg's interest in computer sciences. In order to speed up the testing of blood samples, for example, he developed a machine which tested the sensitivity of bacteria to antibiotics in liquid; the results were recorded in another machine which defused the light by particles. Working with a student physicist, Garst Reese, he developed a series of devices. One reflected needle sensitivities on a meter; a Richter adding machine then printed numbers corresponding to the needles on paper tapes. With tapes applied to walls and using rulers to measure across, the pattern of the bacteria's sensitivity to particular antibiotics could be seen over time. There was a computer center at the University, although not at the medical school, and between midnight and 12:15 a.m. -- the time available on the computer -- Dr. Lindberg could feed the cards (onto which information had been applied) into the computer and get a summary of results. It still took two days to process data from one day's experiments. Despite the Rube Goldberg character of the devices and processes then available, it was obvious that if more sophisticated machinery could be developed, the recording and analysis time could be reduced by extraordinary amounts. Already the rough mechanistic system was much faster than performing each step by hand. It was also more consistent in quality -- the infamous handwriting of physicians and lab personnel always being a problematic factor in assuring accuracy in lab tests.

The experiments brought more support from the university and from outside sources. In short order -- within the first two years of his presence at the University of Missouri -- Dr. Lindberg and Dr. Gwilyn Lodwick developed the first electronic reporting system for use in hospitals. The process became more sophisticated so that the automated testing of blood samples led to mathematical modeling and subsequently to instant feedback. The by-products included the compilation of files on particular cases, both of particular bacteriological strains and their pathological effects, and of particular patients. The new approach also led to an automated billing system.

Thus, a few years later, while the computer science effort was still in its infancy in Missouri, the Regional Medical Program possibility gave this approach to the modernization of health care a boost. One of the distinctive features of the first grant proposal submitted by the Missouri RMP and approved by the Office of Regional Medical Programs was its emphasis on automated information systems and their potential capacity to link bedside to laboratory, and to link small towns to medical centers. Indeed, over the next decade, it was pioneering work in computers and automated information systems on the one hand, and very fundamental training of physicians, nurses, and other health care personnel in intensive care procedures and other lifesaving modes, that made Missouri one of the most prominent of the RMPs.

One special computer program that got national attention involved taking medical histories from patients. This was field tested in the office of Dr. Jack Bass and his private practice in Salem, Missouri. Many were skeptical: Would not persons who were generally unsophisticated, and especially unsophisticated with respect to technology such as personal computers, be intimidated by talking to machines? Actually, in a little informal "control study", Dr. Bass found that people were generally more forthcoming when "punching in" answers posed by a computer than when elaborating their conditions and symptoms and concerns and histories directly to a nurse or physician.[13] This extraordinarily useful lesson, today applied on a wide scale, has made one part of the diagnosis process simpler and more comprehensive, probably without adding cost to that process. More immediately, it brought some fame to Dr. Bass and the Missouri RMP when CBS TV Morning News took its cameras into what quickly became known as "Dr. Mock's Office" to record the pioneering procedure. Parade magazine did a story on the project.[14]

This experiment was followed by others, including computerized searches for symptoms and diagnosis of medical conditions, where individual physicians or other professionals could, through computers, link to base lines of advanced medical and biomedical information.

Another pioneering program was a computerized information bank which facilitated matching heart and kidney patients' vital information (i.e., blood type) with potential organ donors.

In its eight years of actual operations, the Missouri program invested almost $19 million in federal funds in over 100 projects. Some of its programs were very sophisticated. Many were relatively simple. Some helped to develop new technologies from diagnostic capacities to treatment modes. Most did exactly what the authors of the legislation, and the President who inspired it, expected: They brought more doctors, nurses and other health personnel up to speed with advanced knowledge, and so permitted the delivery of that knowledge, through more sophisticated care, to people.

All the hospitals in Missouri and most of the health care professionals in the state were involved in some way or another in the Missouri Regional Medical Program. All the professional associations -- 22 in all, plus the Missouri Farm Bureau Federation and the Missouri Federation of Women's Clubs -- were partners in the enterprise. Most communities in the state participated in some direct way.[15]

As those who developed its RMP are the first to assert, Missouri already had some traditions of cooperation in the health field. The rivalries between medical schools were not overly intense, except perhaps in St. Louis. As a state with strong Democratic and Republican party organizations, bipartisan cooperation was not unheard of. Even the medical doctors and the osteopaths had begun to talk to each other at the time Regional Medical Programs came along. The State Board of Health Registration for the Healing Arts licensed physicians and all other health professionals except, as Dr. Allen notes, Christian Science practitioners, nurses and chiropractors -- which had their own boards.

Underlying the Missouri story is an obvious predilection -- regardless of bureaucracies and specializations and regional differences and rivalries — which was to help people. Also obviously, a group of committed, even enthusiastic individuals from a variety of disciplines joined in a common cause and made the Missouri Regional Medical Program work well.

The exceptional volunteer service rendered by the Regional

Advisory Group was a most important factor in the success of the program. This group, about 50 strong, was representative of producers and consumers of health services in Missouri. Included were a Project Review Committee which concerned itself with the technical merits of proposals, and a Liaison Committee which represented the interests of professional disciplines and special health concerns of consumers.

When the political handwriting on the national wall became visible, suggesting that congressional support for Regional Medical Programs was fading, the Missourians took steps to insure that some of the programs begun under RMP would continue. The University itself invested more in the development of computer systems related to medical diagnosis and treatment and the retrieval of information. The Missouri Kidney Foundation took over programs begun under RMP but which had always benefitted from its own expertise. The Heart Association and Cancer Society did the same. The medical schools did not automatically drop programs just because federal funds from RMP ceased. Community hospitals have gone up and down in their financial fortunes and in populations served, but some programs begun under RMP still continue. Networks expanded under RMP (even if, in the case of this particular state they did not originate with it) still function.

Missouri is not necessarily now, and was perhaps not then, the perfect model of cooperation and medical advance. But it was, in the case of RMP, a model of what a determined group of professionals can do for the people at large if they have a deep concern and a genuine desire to serve.

It was no surprise to those who knew him that, in 1971, Dr. Vernon Wilson should be asked to come to Washington to be administrator of a newly-formed bureau of the U.S. Public Health Service, the Health Services and Mental Health Administration. That Bureau by then housed the Division of Regional Medical Programs.

Notes:

1. Interview with Dr. William Allen, September 1993.

2. Association of American Medical Colleges, Executive Council Meeting Minutes (Open Session), Feb. 6, 1965, p. 6.

3. Much of the information in this chapter, particularly that which is "anecdoted" comes form a series of structural conversations held in Columbia, Mo. in September 1993, arranged for the author by Dr. Arthur Rikli, long-time director of the Missouri Regional Medical Program. Participants included: Jim Watson, Association Dir. MORMP; Fred Frazier, MORMP Information Officer; W.R. Kimel, Dean Emeritus, College of Engineering; Gayle Adams, Professor Emeritus, College of Engineering; Dr. Joye P. Nunn, School of Journalism; Dr. William C. Allen, Professor Emeritus, Dept. of Family and Community Medicine, UM School of Medicine; Dr. Gordon Brown, Chairman, Dept. of Health Service Management; Lloyd Harmon, past Director, American Heart Association of Missouri; and Dr. Wyeth Hamlin, internist and former Chairman, MORMP.

4. Interview with Dr. Allen.

5. Ibid.

6. George Wakerlin, "Missouri Regional Medical Program," Missouri Medicine, Feb. 1967, p. 91.

7. U.S. DHEW, Division of Regional Medical Programs, Directory of Regional Medical Programs, 1969.

8. Columbia conversations, Sept. 1993.

9. Interview with Dr. Allen.

10. Interview with Dr. Wilson conducted by Donald A. B. Lindberg, M.D., July 24, 1991 at the National Library of Medicine., p. 11.

11. Ibid., p. 1.

12. Interview with Dr. Lindberg, Jan. 6, 1994

13. Arthur D Rikli, Fred V. Lucus, Fred Frazier, "The Automated Physicians Assistant," Clinical Engineering News, Feb. 1976. (See also interview with Dr. Rikli conducted by Mr. Storm Whaley, July 25, 1991).

14. "The Automated Physicians Assistant," op. cit.

15. "Ideas, Action, Progress: Cooperation in Health Care," Missouri Regional Medical Program, 1966-71.

Chapter 10

Washington/Alaska

The Washington/Alaska Regional Program covered a vaster expanse than any other in the country. The connection between the two states was natural in two respects, one being simply that Alaska did not have a medical school — a critical element required by the law for delineating a region. The other was historic. There had been, in fact, a long association between the two states. It used to be that almost the only way to get to Alaska almost was through Washington; the ferry service from Seattle to Anchorage was the way most people traveled back and forth. Even the telecommunications system to Alaska was based in Washington. [1]

Montana and Idaho also were without medical schools although their legislatures periodically attempted to get such started, believing that the existence of a medical school gave greater credibility to the economic and intellectual vitality of any state. In short, no self-respecting state should be without a medical school.

Washington's own medical school was a post-World War II phenomenon, begun in 1945. James Haviland, who had been at the medical school since the beginning, recalls that Alaska actually helped create the medical school. Alaska by the 1950's had a surplus of Hill-Burton funds, and somehow arranged to expend some of these in Washington, the justification being that medical care was already, in those days, often being provided for Alaskans by Washington physicians, especially in complicated medical cases.

The rise of the University of Washington Medical School from 1945 to 1965 was extraordinary. It reflected in some ways the rapid expansion of the national medical capacity, including the rapid development of the nation-wide biomedical research enterprise funded largely by the federal government. But the early medical deans, Ed Turner, George Aagaard, John Hogness and Bob VanCitters, in succession seized a variety of opportunities to build a dynamic new institution of national stature, and over two decades, they did so. The development also reflected the leadership of a great university president, Charles Odegaard. Later in this period, it was helpful to have the help of Henry (Scoop) Jackson and Warren Magnuson, the extraordinary team of U.S. Senators from Washington, pushing their state's interest in every arena from the defense and shipbuilding industries to the university and its medical school.

But it was the internal dynamism of the institution that was the more important element. Medical departments were being strengthened one by one, and their chairmen had considerable influence in the running of the institution. A few of them, like the dean and associate deans, had a broad interest in the role of the institution in the region and the nation; and everybody at the medical school wanted to draw on the largest possible person power pool, to fill faculty teaching and clinical positions, and to draw from the largest possible patient population to build up particular treatment and teaching specialties and recruiting students. But no department chairman, as the first Regional Medical Director, Dr. Donal Sparkman remembers, was specifically interested in linking the medical school with particular communities across the state and region. [2]

Dr. Jack Lein, who was on the faculty of the school when RMPs began and now directs public relations for the university, recalls the situation as follows: "Those of us who were involved in medical education spent our lives at the undergraduate level behind the wall of the university, in the medical school behind the wall of the university, took our internship behind the wall of the university, took our residency behind the wall of the university. [We had] then had gone on to the staff of the university to teach people about how to practice medicine... Until this time the relationship of the medical school to the community had been one of sending someone out from a department to a typical medical society meeting, which consisted of 15 martinis, a sumptuous repast, a business meeting, and then a scientific talk for those people who were still awake." [3]

Others represented the university in different ways. Dr. Roy

Schwarz was concerned about the growing if spasmodic rumblings in the Montana and Idaho legislatures that their states needed their own medical school. Somehow he helped to persuade the governments of these adjacent states that it would actually be cheaper to send their best students to the University of Washington medical school than to try to start from scratch and build schools in Boise and Helena. He offered an alternative: Washington would take a number of the best medical school applicants from those states into its medical school, with Idaho and Montana subsidizing the tuition.

Another positive factor that helped in the development of the WARMP was that, in still another instance, the State Medical Society took an interest in it. In contrast to the medical school department chairmen, the practicing physicians of the state were interested in communities across the state, and they were interested in the development of their practices in those communities with help from the medical school. The State Medical Society had already developed a consultative network capacity. Less than many other state medical societies did they feel threatened by new federally supported programs. So they joined with the leaders of the medical school creating Washington/Alaska RMP.

Of course Washington dominated the bi-state program. But from the beginning when Dr. VanCitters called his friend the governor of Alaska and asked him to appoint somebody to help develop the connection, that connection was strong. Yet aside from the call from the university to the governor's office in Juneau, the governors of the two states were not involved.

Dr. Hogness and Dr. VanCitters thought it would be useful to bring in an outsider, Dr. Donal Sparkman, to run the program, believing, apparently correctly, that an outsider would be less threatening to a department chairman and to other, more conservative members of the school faculty than would someone from within the university.

As in other programs, in Washington there was an early strong emphasis on continuing education. Some of the component programs were novel. Not all of them, however. For example, although they were sophisticated in their production and packaging of 25-minute videotapes, sending them around to county medical societies and other institutions did not prove especially effective as a means of continuing medical education.

On the other hand, a preceptor program begun by Dr. Lein proved to be one of the most important of all the programs. It did not cost much, and it did satisfy both promising young physicians in communities distant from the university and provide, through them, links to those communities. Ted Phillips was a young physician who had gone to Sitka, Alaska with the Indian Health Service and was in private practice when Don Sparkman, newly appointed director of the Washington/Alaska Regional Medical Program, made a trip to Juneau, then down through southeastern Alaska, to see what the needs were. Young Dr. Phillips was impressed that a physician from the medical school would actually come to his neck of the woods to ask such questions. He thought he was already practicing pretty good medicine. He had somehow heard about the DeBakey report, and the notion of establishing a small handful of centers of medical excellence from which information would flow, out to Sitka and its equivalent communities across the length and breadth of the country, seemed to him pretty presumptuous. He gave Dr. Sparkman his view of needs and the quality of existing practice in his community. Later, feeling more comfortable with the Seattle program, he took an opportunity for preceptorship to come down "to learn how to put in a pacemaker." [4] Thus was recruited one of the School of Medicine's most popular and effective faculty members who, in less than three years, was to come back to Seattle to be Chairman of the Department of Family Medicine.

John Hogness, by then Vice-President for Medical Affairs and his successor, Bob VanCitters, then Dean of the Medical School, continued their efforts. Dr. Hogness persisted in encouraging county medical leaders as well as the state medical society to join, acting in solidifying the new program. [5] Drs. Hogness, Vancitters and Sparkman quickly enlisted thirty other health professionals to join the Regional Advisory Board to direct the effort. As it became clear that the planning grant would probably be approved, it was urgent that representatives of the two states identify their needs. The first planning grant for the program came in September of 1966. The usual studies and pilot programs were begun and on February 1, 1968, the WARMP went into full action. [6]

A preceptorship program proved a success in all ways. Operating for most of the decade of WARMP, an average of 50 physicians per year came from communities all across the two states to train in hospitals of Seattle, Spokane and Takoma. [7] The community physicians joined a physician specialist on his rounds and incorporated what they learned into their practice. The result was several hundred practicing physicians who were much more expert in treating the important chronic diseases, especially heart and other cardiovascular diseases, cancer and stroke.

In an unusual extension of the traditional postgraduate preceptorships, WARMP also established one for nurses in conjunction with the Harborview Medical Center. In this case, nurses from rural areas of Montana and Idaho as well as Washington and Alaska followed a similar program, except that the areas they focused on were more varied, extending from dialysis to emergency room to pediatrics, orthopedics, anesthesia, and obstetrics to intensive care. There was even a preceptorship established in radiation physics which, along with other training programs, ultimately resulted in the creation of the Northwest Medical Physics Center at the University of Washington. This center in turn assisted in the development of 28 radiation therapy facilities across the two-state area.

The Alaska Health Sciences Library -- "the first such reference center in that state" -- was another early project of WARMP, with other funding coming from the Public Health Service. The library filled an enormous gap; within a few years, the library was being patronized by 80% of the physicians in that state, a much higher usage than the national average.[8]

The needs and opportunities in health care delivery across the landscape of Washington from the eastern, sparsely-populated areas to the big cities, and throughout Alaska, were so great that it seemed easy to find opportunities to carry out the intent of the Heart Disease, Cancer and Stroke Act of 1965. Given the central need for continuing education, WARMP's Information Education Support Unit was among its more active elements. For example, from 1968 to 1973, 62 continuing education programs were produced, utilizing physicians or specialists from the University of Washington faculty and the community and the technical facilities of a local television firm. Aside from the questionable effectiveness of sending out videotapes, what did seem to work was the airing of these programs on education television. [9]

Regional cooperative arrangements in the two states were fostered. With the Washington State Hospital Association, WARMP developed a consortium of 18 institutions in the central part of the state, which shared in-service education programs and a range of other resources. With the Washington State Medical Association, the School of Medicine and several county medical societies, WARMP surveyed almost 4,800 physicians about their continuing education needs in heart, cancer and stroke, with a 79% response rate. A program was developed on the basis of these needs and preferences. [10]   In western Washington, 10 community hospitals, typically with 30-40 beds, joined to form a Health Services Consortium which linked Virginia Mason Hospital in Seattle (with 300 beds) and a range of special expertise to the needs of 10 community hospitals. This program was deemed so successful by those outside as well as those participating in it that at the end of RMP, it was continued by the Kellogg Foundation. [11]

In central Washington a subregional medical center was established in Yakima, once more focusing in significant part on cardiology, although extending to other fields. The strengthened capacity so attracted physicians that the Director of the Program, Dr. Jack Gufstafson, subsequently reported that in a period when other nonurban areas in the state were losing physicians, 11 new physicians moved into the Yakima area during the first two years of this program. [12]

The leaders of the Washington/Alaska Program decided to deal directly with the problems of diverse populations within the region. Even before such an emphasis was supported by the Nixon Administration, they initiated or supported programs directed at the problems of Native Americans in Alaska, in reservations in the State of Washington and among Indian populations in urban centers. They worked with the Urban League to test for hypertension in inner-city blacks. They also directed attention to the increasing number of Hispanic residents of the area and of health problems of migrant workers. They helped to bring together leaders of the Alaskan tribes to form a health network, and trained Native Alaskans as health workers. Of the 162 projects approved and supported during the decade, 17 were directly and exclusively concerned with minority health problems, and many more had components which addressed such needs.[13]

This is especially impressive given that there were also 17 programs dealing with cardiovascular diseases, ten dealing with cancer problems, 12 with geriatric care, and seven with kidney diseases. The programs in continuing education reinforced this pattern; as a general proposition, cardiovascular problems were at the center of many of them.

Spending about $2 million per year to serve a region with a population of 4 million, the Washington/Alaska Program illuminated the landscape of need, and demonstrated across a wide spectrum how those needs could be met. As in many other cases, those involved in the WARMP believed it was important and successful. But aside from the enthusiasm of the participants, there is another clue about success which may be even stronger. An extraordinary number of programs begun under the WARMP continued after the program went out of existence. One of the more prominent ones was Seattle's "Medic One," which began as a mobile coronary care unit, operated by the Seattle Fire Department under the supervision at Harborview Medical Center. It was succeeded by 10 smaller, neighborhood-based vehicles which covered the city's ninety square miles and population of a half million, responding to all. When the closing of RMP meant a cutoff of federal funds, there was, Dr. Sparkman remembers, "a backlash of criticism of the donors." But a newspaper-sponsored fund drive and assistance from the Rotary Club filled the gap, and the city subsequently put the program in its own budget to the tune of more than $1 million a year. Meanwhile, WARMP had trained scores of firemen, in 1,000 hour training sessions -- a good thing, for by 1973 the annual emergency calls to Medic One went up to 18,000. [14]

The University took over some programs, the State some, the Washington State Heart Association adopted several; Urban Leagues in several cities, the VA hospital in a few cases, private foundations and federal agencies took over others. As many as 20% of the programs that had begun as demonstration projects were carried forward by others when Regional Medical Programs went out of existence. [15]

Still, it may have been in other ways that the program made its greatest difference. At the end of the decade, the University of Washington School of Medicine was very much involved in communities across the two states. "Subregional" networks of health care training and providing institutions had been established. Continuing education for physicians, nurses, and other allied health workers had become highly visible. In this period some 100 persons -- physicians, nurses, allied health personnel and lay citizens -- had joined in regular sessions of the RMP Advisory Group to address problems and make decisions about health care in Washington and Alaska.

Notes:

1. Interviews with Dr. Donal Sparkman and Mr. James Haviland, September, 1993. Additional general information and commentary comes from conversations with Dr. John Hogness, Dr. Robert Petersdorf, Dr. Augustus Swenson and Dr. Ted Phillips, in August and September 1993.
2. Interview with Dr. Sparkman.
3. "Minutes of the Last RAB Meeting, May 15, 1976,11 Washington/Alaska Regional Medical Program, June 10, 1976, p. 13.
4. Ibid., p. 14.
5. Interview with Dr. Hogness.
6. U.S. DHEW, Division of Regional Medical Programs, Directory of Regional Medical Programs, 1969.
7. "W/ARMP in Retrospect, 1968-1976,11 Washington/Alaska Regional Medical Program, pp. 75-76. See also interviews with Dr. Sparkman' and Mr. Haviland; and "Minutes of the Last' RAB Meeting," op. cit., p. 14.
8. Ibid., pp. 83-83. See also "Minutes of the Last RAB Meeting;" op. cit., Dr. Jack Lien achieved instant notoriety for himself, the new library and W/ARMP when television cameras and the Associated Press reported his opening line at the dedication ceremony in the winter of 1969: "I've closed a lot of bars in my life but this is the first time I've opened a library."
9. "W/ARMP in Retrospect," pp. 56-57.
10. Ibid., p. 63.
11. Ibid., pp. 85-86.
12. Ibid. pp. 74-75.
13. Ibid., pass. (author's calculations).
14. Ibid., introduction and project description, p. 40.
15. Ibid. (author's calculations).

Chapter 11

California

Some of the bitterest opposition to the DeBakey Commission and its proposals came from the Medical Society of Los Angeles County. Some of the strongest support for Regional Medical Programs, as it was described and defined by law, came from leaders of the medical schools of Southern California and leaders of state health agencies. No state in the country has as many socio-political fault lines as California. They reach far beyond the old economic competition of San Francisco and Los Angeles and beyond the general rivalry between of Northern California and Southern California. In 1965, almost 20 million people lived in California. The population was served by an extraordinary system of higher education and, as a part of that, by eight medical schools. The latter fact helped to persuade Californians with different views about the new program to give it a try.

In 1966, Dr. Roger Egeberg was the new dean of the school of medicine at the University of Southern California. The RMP national director, Dr. Robert Marston, had come to town to talk about the Program. While a new medical care initiative out of Washington, D.C. was the last thing on Dr. Egeberg's mind -- "Washington could have been in Siberia as far as my thinking was concerned" -- there were two things about the description of possibilities Dr. Marston offered that were intriguing.[1] The first was that California itself should decide how to organize the region, and the second was that the law encouraged medical schools to reach out into adjacent and even distant communities to build archipelagos of action which would extend the best medical information and techniques to local physicians and facilities.[2]

Dr. Egeberg was not the only one who had been troubled by the fact that in smaller towns and cities across California there were "still quite a few doctors practicing who had graduated from medical schools which had long since become extinct because they didn't rate. So there was a worry about the level of health care."[3] In all, he thought the new programs sounded like a good idea.

However "the university was conservative about it; the faculty was, but the executive committee, after I explained it to them, came along. So we were the first people in California to join." [4] UCLA was one of the next. Dr. Donald F. Brayton, Associate Dean of UCLA's School of Medicine, joined in the local conversation. Both deans sought out friends in the California Medical Association, and conversations steadily expanded. [5]

Paul Ward, who was to become Executive Director of the California Committee on Regional Medical Programs, thought his state had been relatively slow in organizing. After all, the first group to talk about such possibility had sat down together in the fall of 1965, before the law was signed by President Johnson; they met infrequently for more than a year and they did receive a planning grant of $223,000 in November of 1966.[6] During this period the California Medical Association and the California Hospital Administration were very much involved in the conversation and agreed to be a part of the program, and of the organization administering the program. That organization, the California Committee on Regional Medical Programs, would be composed of: the deans of the eight medical schools and the two schools of public health in the state; representatives of the California Medical Association and the Hospital Association; the Director of the State Department of Public Health, representatives from the California Heart Association and the California Division of the American Cancer Society, as well as eight persons representing the general public.[7]

In April 1967, the California Committee on Regional Medical Programs received its first supplemental award to begin active planning for regional medical activities. It allocated its funds to the medical schools of University of Southern California, UCLA, Loma Linda University and the University of California at San Francisco, and to the California Medical Association and the California Hospital Association. By October 1967, four other medical schools were funded for their planning round:

UC-Davis, Stanford, UC-San Diego and the California College of Medicine.[8]

Thus was the entire State covered, with regions centered on medical schools, and with all major players, including the California Medical Association, actively involved in the planning. Most of the schools put strong persons in charge of their efforts. It was a special advantage to have Paul Ward as Executive Director. He had served in Governor Edmund C. Brown's administration in the State for seven of its eight years. For much of that time he was Administrator of the Health and Welfare Agency of the State which included the Departments of Public Health, Rehabilitation, Hygiene and Social Welfare. Indeed, he was a member of the governor's cabinet and, perhaps more importantly, a long-time friend and confident of Pat Brown. He was available to take the new RMP job because Governor Pat Brown had just been replaced by Governor Ronald Reagan.

The Chairman of the California Committee remained the positive and affable Roger Egeberg, a man of extraordinary energy and warmth, who had at one point been personal physician to General Douglas MacArthur in the Pacific campaign. A big man with a big heart, whose sometimes gruff approach was always belied by twinkling eyes and a hearty laugh, he had been in the vanguard of California health leaders who favored RMP. It was natural that he was asked to be Chairman of the Committee.

It was not the only committee he chaired in Los Angeles, or in the State or in the university world. He always insisted on clarity and straightforwardness and had in the course of one meeting demanded that members of the Committee stop using acronyms: "Goddamn it," he said, "stop using initials. I don't know what this CCRMC is that you keep talking about." Paul Ward replied, "Roger, it is the California Committee on Regional Medical Programs of which you have been the Chair for the last two years."[9]

Even within the medical school-centered California subregions the challenge was awesome. For example, Dr. Pettit of USC, who directed the program based in that institution's School of Medicine, recorded that in 1965 the area encompassed by Region 5 was approximately 3,400 square miles and had a population of 4,385,000. He commented: "Most of this territory is highly urbanized and is highly urbanized is beset by all the health care problems characteristic of modern American cities."[10] The same was certainly of the UCLA Region, Region 4. There was a great contrast in Region 6, headquartered at the School of Medicine at Loma Linda University and Region 2, headquartered at the University of California Davis. They had more diverse populations and by far more rural populations in their borders. Each of them had a Nevada city and area in their territory, Reno being connected to UC-Davis and Las Vegas to Loma Linda.

The demarcation lines were recognized from the outset as being arbitrary. Some were clearly so, but that would have to be worked out later. For example, along old Highway US 99, "some doctors in Redding would prefer to look for advice and help to UC-Davis; others also in Redding would rather look to UC-San Francisco." [11] So the needs and preferences of the local physicians were sought and a practical approach would be evolved. For example, "It may well turn out that the practitioners and hospitals would want to make cooperative arrangements on cardiovascular disease with Davis, and on cancer with San Francisco." [12]

The early programs supported by the California Regional Medical Program all seemed sensible, fundamental and straightforward. They included: "1) A review of all available mortality and morbidity data collected in California. 2) An analysis of all discharges from all hospitals in the state by diagnosis, age, sex and geographic origin of patients. 3) An inventory of advanced clinical resources in California available to take care of patients with heart disease, cancer and stroke. 4) An inventory and analysis of training programs for health fields other than medicine. 5) Interviews with practicing physicians to determine resources and patterns of referral used for patients with heart disease, cancer and stroke." [13]

Also from an early date there was a special effort to link community hospitals to the library resources of the university medical libraries. The first arrangement between the UCLA Biomedical Library and the Library at the Fresno Hospital was in fact a three-way arrangement. If the UCLA Library could not immediately provide information requested by physicians through the Fresno Library, UCLA's "TWX" linkage with the National Library of Medicine in Bethesda was put into play. This meant, for example, that all information available through Medlars was, for the first time, available to Fresno. [14]

Naturally, continuing education for physicians, nurses, and other health professions was considered key to the entire enterprise. But in the early days, it was not an automatic application of particular forms of continuing education. Or at least, not in Roger Egeberg's experience. He arranged for groups of Bakersfield physicians and surgeons to come into the city and attend lectures by USC physicians on the teaching staff. The response was underwhelming. So the reverse was tried. Teams of the USC physicians went to Bakersfield, at the request of that hospital's department chairs, and created teaching clinics there. This worked. [15]

The change in the national administration came in January 1969. Richard Nixon had narrowly defeated Hubert Humphrey the previous November, and Democrats feared the worst, feeling certain that Nixon would move immediately to dismantle Great Society programs. Yet he did not. Instead, as will be spelled out subsequently, the new administration moved cautiously on the domestic policy front -- in significant part because the Democrats still controlled Congress. The RMP statute had already been renewed for three years before the end of the Johnson Administration. It was renewed again, with the Nixon Administration underway, in 1970.

About the time of the first congressional renewal, RMP's critics in California, including those in the California Academy of General Practice, noted with concern the "accommodations" many in the medical community were making to new arrangements inspired by this federal initiative. Wrote Dr. Wilfred Snodgrass: "On reviewing the law's brief three year history, it is extraordinary how peaceably RMP has settled over the medical community."[16] He seemed to see in RMP a Trojan horse. That was a real danger.

Among other things RMP is slowly moving to the establishment of national standards with the coercive compliance compelled by such standards... The infiltration into organized medicine is now so complete that the voice of the California RMP areas have, by default, become the voice of California medicine. No conquest was ever more complete or bloodless.[17]

As in other regions and as time went on the California Regional Medical Program could justifiably point with pride to a range of successful programs. One extraordinary set of initiatives in the metropolitan areas was a series of programs focused on low-income communities inhabited principally by minority groups. Not only were community programs organized but in fact a post-graduate medical school was established.

An RMP grant undergirded the first three years of recruitment and program development of the Charles R. Drew Postgraduate Medical School, named for "the eminent Negro surgeon who pioneered blood plasma research and blood banking." [18] The school was to be -- and did become -- the academic arm of the Los Angeles County/Martin Luther King Jr. General Hospital completed in 1971. Together they served the predominantly black and predominantly poor L.A. communities of Watts and Willowbrook. The school and hospital were given responsibility for this area of the city, delineated as RMP Area IX, serving a population of about 500,000 persons. [19]

In east Los Angeles, the UCLA medical school set up special task force to assess and begin to meet health needs in a barrio serving basically a Hispanic population. Another program was focused on primary care for Native Americans living in a particular section of Los Angeles. Most of these programs had O.E.O. funds and often other federal funds. But many of them were funded as well -- and sometimes first -- by Regional Medical Programs.

The emphasis on poorer and in many cases minority populations in large metropolitan areas was natural. The high incidence of hypertension and heart disease among low-income blacks was already beginning to be a matter of national attention, and the early programs focused on this even as they helped to build service connections between the teaching hospitals and the communities in Los Angeles, San Diego, San Francisco and other cities. The straightforward insistence of the Nixon administration on elevating the needs of the poor who did not have medical care coverage accelerated the trend, at least in California.

By 1973 -- even as reviews about the future of the national program were being undertaken in more critical veins -- the California program and its medical school principals were responding actively to the evolving need. As CCRMP moved into the new era, Paul Ward seemed to take special pleasure in the new emphasis. In an article in California Medicine appearing in April 1973 but written earlier, Paul Ward stated with pleasure and optimism: "Partnerships now developing among community and professional interests could lead to significantly better quality of health care available for all our citizens and a gratifying improvement in the health care delivery system." [20]

Some Californians in Washington were not so sanguine. Other of Ward's compatriots had left government service; for example, Secretary Bob Finch had been eased out of his job in June 1970 after eighteen months, and the versatile, redoubtable Elliot Richardson, skilled in the ways of politics and bureaucracy, become Secretary. Richardson had no animus toward the program; in fact, it seemed like a reasonable effort to him. But there were increasingly serious budgetary concerns and, regardless of who was responsible for the gradual diversification of program, hence the dilution of original purpose of RMPs, it seemed difficult to sum up what they had accomplished across the country or even in California. [21]

Notes:

1. Interview with Dr. Egeberg, conducted by Diane Rehn, July 30, 1991, National Library of Medicine, p. 5.
2. Ibid., pp. 5-6.
3. ibid., p. 6.
4. Ibid.
5. Donald F. Brayton, "UCLA Regional Medical Programs: Present and Future," Bulletin of the Los Angeles County Medical Society, Nov. 1967.
6. Paul D. Ward, "A Progress Report on Heart Disease, Cancer and Stroke," Bulletin of the Los Angeles County Medical Society, Nov 1967, p. 16.
7. Ibid.
8. Ibid.
9. Rehm interview with Dr. Egeberg, op. cit., p. 10.
10. Donald W. Petit, "Area I, California Regional Medical Programs at USC," Bulletin of the Los Angeles County Medical Society, Dec. 1967, p. 16.
11. Paul D. Ward, op. cit. p. 17.
12. Ibid.
13. Ibid.
14. Donald F. Brayton, op. cit., p. 23.
15. Interview with Dr. Egeberg.
16. Wilfred Snodgras, "The Changing Philosophy in Regional Medical Programs," Bulletin of the Los Angeles County Medical Society," August 7, 1969, p. 18.
17. Ibid., p. 20.
18. Mitchell W. Spellman, "Drew Postgraduate Medical School," Bulletin of the

Los Angeles County Medical Society, June 17, 1971.

19. Ibid.

20. Paul D. Ward, "Regional Medical Programs," California Medicine, April 1973.

21. See Interview with Dr. John Zapp. Dr. Zapp says that Secretary Richardson felt that it was increasingly difficult to present convincing evidence to the office of Management and Budget that the RMP program was worthwhile. In conversations with the author in 1992, Mr. Richardson stressed that the principal factors in changing policy were the changing demographic and economic context in the early 1970's and the evolving views of experts from a variety of fields on what was needed to improve the health status of Americans.

Chapter 12

Political Transition, Program Developments

It was really no surprise when the provisions of the Heart Disease, Cancer and Stroke Amendments of 1965, and the Regional Medical Programs they authorized, were extended with no great difficulty in October 1968 (Public Law 90-547). What may be surprising to some is that Regional Medical Programs were also extended with little difficulty at the behest of the Nixon Administration and its first Secretary of the Department of Health Education and Welfare, Robert Finch, in 1970. [1] The new administration did push for the removal of categorical programs and wanted to add prevention and rehabilitation to the original specified categories of activity: research, training, diagnosis and, in demonstration form, treatment. Dr. Roger Egeberg, by then Assistant Secretary for Health and Scientific Affairs, and Dr. Michael DeBakey were among the principal witnesses testifying on the cluster of bills, (finally included in the aggregate Health Services Act of 1970), dealing with these questions.

In its collective wisdom, Congress added kidney diseases to the existing categorical list in addition to those features proposed by the new team at HEW. It also authorized increasing annual expenditures for RMP: $125 million in 1970, $150 million in 1971 and $250 million for fiscal year 1972. [2] These figures were significantly below the original estimates by the Johnson Administration as to where the programs would be fiscally at the end of six years. And, the figures were below those authorized by the Congress for Comprehensive Health Planning; the Administration, with congressional agreement, gave CHP a funding ceiling of more than twice that authorized for RMP. Also added into the comprehensive measure was the National Center for Health Services Research and Development.

From the beginning of the Nixon administration, with the Democrats still in control of Congress, the struggle over organizational, programmatic and budgetary initiatives was a constant element in what is called the governmental process. Time after time committees of Congress, or individual members, proposed new national attacks on newly identified priorities. They proposed the addition of new institutes, program categories for established institutes, or at least changes of names in institutes, of NIH. In almost every instance, the administration resisted. Time after time, Congress added funds to categorized program budgets. In every case save one, the administration opposed.

The great exception, of course, was the National Cancer Act of 1971. Otherwise a succession of Secretaries of Health, Education and Welfare, and especially Assistant Secretaries for Health, went marching up the Hill to urge restraint instead of expansion, consolidation instead of proliferation, holding the line instead of busting the budget.

Those in charge of Health, Education and Welfare in the Nixon years were not simply reactionary. Nixon's first Secretary of HEW, Bob Finch and his Undersecretary, Jack Venneman, produced a White Paper which many accepted as a coherent approach to a federal role in health and which was followed for the next several years. In developing it, one source of expertise and judgment they relied on was the career Civil Service, or at least a significant number of key individuals in the federal service, who in the best tradition shared their knowledge and judgment objectively and forthrightly.

The debates about principles, goals, and priorities were spasmodic in their sequence and dispersed as to the arenas in which they were held. But they were, in the main, rational and civil. Karl Yordy, a long-time civil servant who helped to organize the RMP program in 1965, remembers thinking, when he was first introduced to the Nixon Health Team headed by Secretary Finch, that these were intelligent, high-minded, reasonable people. His subsequent encounters over the next several years did not dissuade him from that view; indeed, they reinforced it. [3]

The 1970's presented a new array of national health needs. Principal among them was the rising cost of health care which, added to the persistent pattern of impoverished minorities, seemed to raise the problem of access to medical care to a more urgent level. [4] Medical care costs, pushed upward in significant part by the Medicare budget, suggested to many persons that Dr. Paul Ellwood was right in recommending that the government support the development of health maintenance organizations, in order to get ahead of the health cost curve and to address the need for proactive, preventive care. The number of physicians trained with federal help during the preceding decade increased by more than 60 thousand, but the problem of "geographical distribution" was as severe as ever. New means of persuading physicians to go to underserved areas were required. In the administration's view, a central problem of the '60s, scarce hospital beds, had become just the reverse: how to control the proliferation of unneeded beds. Hence its proposal that Hill-Burton authority be restricted to renovations and not new constructions. With respect to all the above, the Nixon administration sought to strengthen health planning agencies, indeed to use the system of health planning agencies to move towards an opposite goal from that originally intended in the Johnson years, namely to contain the expansion of facilities and technical resources, and in this way to control health costs.

Rationalization of federal programs was an overriding emphasis. The management side was given a special boost when the President proposed reorganizing and renaming the Bureau of the Budget, making it the Office of Management and Budget. Opposition in Congress did not prove formidable and the reorganization plan which redesignated BOB as OMB went into effect in May 1970. [5]

On other issues of contention, Congress did prevail. The President vetoed the extension of the Hill-Burton Act because the bill authorized direct grants which were $350 million in excess of his budget request for 1971 and because it authorized the construction of more new hospitals rather than, as the administration preferred, limiting Hill-Burton grants to modernizing existing facilities. Congress overrode the President's veto on Hill-Burton, the first successful override of a presidential veto in a decade. [6]

Congress and the administration jousted about national health insurance as well as Hill-Burton but agreed on other things, including a program to encourage the development of health maintenance organizations and revisions in health and allied health manpower. But, to repeat, there was no great controversy between the administration and Congress about Regional Medical Programs. The fifty-six programs and the Regional Medical Programs Service thought they had a new lease on life.

When the traditional annual meeting of Regional Medical Programs took place in January 1972, the newest Assistant Secretary of Health and Scientific Affairs, Dr. Merlin K. Duval, Jr., recently Dean of the Medical School of University of Arizona, was upbeat about the administration's health programs and policies, and seemed to imply broad agreement with Congress on a variety of fundamental issues.

> There is little reason to doubt that we are now beginning to move in the proper direction. The right of all citizens to have equal opportunity for good medical care is no longer contested. Nor is there any remaining controversy about a need to control medical costs; to redistribute and maximize the use of existing manpower; and to do all this, and perhaps more, without delay.[7]

The College of Medicine at the University Arizona had been the grantee organization for the Arizona Regional Medical Program, and Dr. Duval had been very positive about RMP. The Arizona program had moved slowly, taking considerable time to bring the physicians of the State on board, a process in which Dr. Duval helped significantly. Ultimately, the President of the Arizona Medical Society, Dr. Richard O. Flynn, became one of the Arizona Program's staunchest advocates. He too had worked to explain to his fellow physicians what the Regional Medical Program was or, "more important, what it wasn't, i.e., a federally dominated program to be stuffed down our throat." [8]

Dr. Duval had even been sanguine about the complementarity of RMP and comprehensive health planning, specifying that they were not in conflict. He thought it especially sensible that his State had named all the members of the Regional Advisory Group for RMP to membership on the Advisory Planning Council for Comprehensive Health Planning and "thus assured complete interdigitation of these two programs." [9]

The newest RMP Director, Dr. Harold Margulies, found a synthesis between the persistent Nixon administration position against the categorical emphasis of RMP – in the legislation it submitted in 1970, in White Papers on Health Policy in 1971 and 1972 -- and ultimate congressional refusal to do away with such emphasis. In the 1972 Factbook on RMP, the balance was presented: "Though RMP continues to have a categorical emphasis, to be effective that emphasis must frequently be subsumed within or made subservient to broader and more comprehensive approaches. RMP must relate primary care to specialized care, affect manpower distribution and utilization, and generally improve the system for delivering comprehensive care." [10]

There were 56 Regional Medical Programs in operation in 1972, one more than the figure of 55 cited in 1970. But there were some changes among the mix. For example, Delaware was given its own regional program in response to increasing agitation on the part of the Delaware Medical Society which was fed up with the domination of Philadelphia's six medical schools in the greater Delaware Valley Regional Medical Program.

It should have been clear, the Delaware doctors thought, that the creation of regions "where three sets of state laws have to be satisfied only impedes progress in the masses of weighty administrative forces." [11] Why not let the State of Delaware itself be a Regional Medical Program? It was, as a State, "ideal for a pilot study in any field of federal government inquiry, be it medicine, economics, law or social services. We have a easy relationship with our State government, and a cross-section of human forces from the ghetto to the farms, from the metropolitan areas to the hamlets, from the very wealthy to the very impoverished and even from the very vocal to the silent majority." [12] The vocal doctors won and in the spring of 1972, the Delaware Regional Medical Program was awarded its first organizational grant as a separate program. Delaware was "once more free to act through the sovereignty of its state." [13] And not through a multi-state regional program.

Similarly, what had been first organized as the Nebraska-South Dakota RMP was divided into two separate programs in 1971. On the other hand, two Ohio programs, that based at the Ohio State University College of Medicine in Columbus and that the Northeast Ohio RMP based in Cleveland at Case Western Reserve, were joined together. [14]

Of the 56 programs, 34 encompassed single states and four encompassed two or more states. Eleven programs were "subregional," usually metropolitan areas within single states. Seven RMPs, most based in major metropolitan areas, extended across state lines. The latter included several of the New York programs, the Memphis Bi-State Program, the Ohio Valley RMP, and the California RMP with two of its subregions including cities in Nevada. [15] Thirteen of the programs served populations of over five million people, twelve served one to three million people, and thirteen included populations of three to five million. Six programs served populations of less than a million. [16]

In 1972, the California RMP was receiving $10 million, the highest level of any RMP in the country. Little Delaware, newly independent, received the least funds that year, approximately $200 thousand. In that seventh year of the program, most of the RMPs, 29, were receiving between $1-2.5 billion a year, with the median funding level cited at $1 million. [17]

Appropriations continued to run way behind authorizations. In fiscal years 1970 and 1971, the first fiscal years controlled by the Nixon administration, the appropriations came closer to matching the authorizations, and the amounts awarded for grants closer to matching the appropriation figure, than in the previous four years. In 1972, $150 million had been authorized (in the extension of the legislation in 1970); $90 million was appropriated and over $110 million actually awarded for grants. [18]

Of the grantee agencies which received the funds and "fiscally administered" programs, 33 were universities or components thereof and 23 were other entities, including 16 new agencies or corporations created especially for this purpose. [19]

In 1972, 2,667 U.S. citizens participated as members of regional advisory groups governing their Regional Medical Programs. Of these, 67% were "providers" and 25% "consumers." Of the provider group, 32% were practicing physicians and a majority of the others were from related health sciences. The average staff for the programs was 25 -- down from an average of 28 in 1969; and of the staff only ten percent were physicians in 1972, down from 15% in 1969. [20]

Although not highlighted in the legislative consideration of the program, minority populations were a new focus. In fiscal year 1972, activities directed at special target populations such as African Americans, Spanish Americans, and Indians more than doubled, from 46 projects in $5.4 million to 147 projects with $17 million in RMP funding. This was a theme across the country. The Michigan RMP began screening Black children for sickle-cell anemia in Grand Rapids. The New Mexico RMP established clinics for Native Americans in the northern part of the State. Most of the metropolitan-based programs increased their focus on minority populations, and Washington, Alaska, and California expanded their emphases. [21]

There were other new emphases. One of them was evaluation. The Director of the RMP Service must have taken pride in reporting that 53 of the 56 RMPs, in 1972, had Evaluation Directors, most of them professionally trained. [22] There was concern about the actual authority of Regional Advisory groups or councils. In the latter connection, there was considerable worry on the part of the staff reviewing the Northeastern Ohio RMP because all power seemed to reside in the twelve-person Executive Committee, most of whom were associated with Case Western Reserve Medical School, rather than with the 55-member Advisory Group. Naturally, a group that large would have made decisions cumbersome, but the staff recommended a reduction in size and greater diversity, specifically so that it would not be so dominated by physicians and there would be more consumer representation. [23] The fundamental point was that it was the Regional Advisory Group, not any committee thereof, that had authority and responsibility for the development of the program and for particular decisions with respect to projects. The latter was important in another connection: An effort was being made to further decentralize decision making, giving individual RMPs and especially their governing authorities, the RAGs, more leeway in decision making.

There was renewed emphasis of an established policy. That policy was that RMP support of projects should usually end after a three-year period, although an allowance of up to two years more could be made in order to ensure the orderly termination of an enterprise or the assumption of its operation by other organizations. The national office must have put considerable pressure on the programs in 1971 in this regard. In that year, only about 40% of RMP initiated operational programs were said to have been ended within the specified time limit. A year later that figure had risen to 75-80 percent. As if building a case for future policy, 1972 report suggested that "roughly 60% of those projects from which RMP grant support is being withdrawn will be continued from other sources at approximately 80% of their RMP funding level. [24]

There were seemingly continuous organizational changes and

leadership changes that had to be contended with. On other health policy fronts, there were also new developments, some of them major, which could easily affect the shape and direction of Regional Medical Programs. The National Cancer Act of 1971, represented a triumph by an unusual alliance -- once more inspired by Mary Lasker – that of President Nixon and Senator Ted Kennedy. The statute had not only given the National Cancer Institute equal status with the combined components of NIH (although this was later reversed) and greatly increased its budget. It also had given NCI a specific mandate to carry out cancer demonstration projects of a wide variety across the country.

The next year, the National Heart Institute -- now the National Heart, Blood and Lung Institute -- was given similar authority, once more with significantly increased funds. The Administration and its Department of Health, Education and Welfare did not oppose the basic proposition outright. But Assistant Secretary Monty Duval expressed reservations about the bill as passed by the Senate on several grounds. For one thing the proposed special authority for the National Heart and Lung Institute to establish 15 cardiovascular and 15 pulmonary centers for basic and clinic research training, as well as 12 model cardiovascular disease prevention clinics, would duplicate what Regional Medical Programs already had authority to do. [25]

Notes:

1. See "Conference Report on Regional Medical Programs and Comprehensive Health Planning and Services Act of 1970," Report no. 91-1590, U.S. House of Representatives, 91st Congress, 2nd Session.
2. Ibid., p. 2.
3. Interviews with Karl Yordy, August 1993.
4. The statements made in this and subsequent paragraphs are easily documentable, but the author has not referenced all of them point by point. Rather he has relied on his own experience as a health policy analyst and commentator during this period, as a founding faculty member of the Health Policy Program (later Health Policy Institute) of the University of California, San Francisco, where he served from 1972 to 1977. He also reviewed this period with David K. Lelewer, a White House Fellow who served both with Secretaries Wilbur Cohen in the Johnson Administration and Bob Finch of the Nixon Administration.
5. Dept. of Health, Education, and Welfare, Office of the Director, NIH, "Legislative Developments" prepared for NIH Advisory Councils, Oct. 14, 1970,

p. 53.

6. Ibid., p. 36.

7. DHEW, Division of Regional Medical Programs Service, "Regional Medical Programs Fact Book," 1972, (Foreword).

8. Richard 0. Flynn, M.D., "Regional Medical Program," Arizona Medicine, 1973 May 30 (5), p. 343.

9. Monty K. Duval, M.D., "Regional Medical Program," Arizona Medicine, 1969 May.

10. "Regional Medical Programs Fact Book," op. cit., p. 4.

11. R. J. Bishoff, M.D., "President's Page," Delaware Medicine, April 1971.

12. Ibid.

13. Ibid.

14. "Regional Medical Programs Fact Book," op. cit., p. 8.

15. Ibid., pp. 6-7.

16. ibid., P. 8.

17. Ibid.

18. Ibid., p. 4.

19. Ibid., p. 10.

20. Ibid., p. 11-12.

21. Ibid., p. 27, (See also Chapters on Washington/Alaska and California).

22. Ibid., p. 29.

23. Ibid.

24. Ibid.

25. "Legislative Developments," op. cit., pp. 3-4.

Chapter 13

Policy Struggle, Death Knell

From an early point in the history of Regional Medical Programs, an organized constituency of recipient organizations came together in traditional American fashion. In fact, the National Association of Regional Medical Programs had its origins in the first meeting of directors and advisors of such programs called by Surgeon General Bill Stewart and RMP Director Bob Marston in January 1967. The meeting's purpose was to start building support for the renewal of the authorizing legislation the next year.

That meeting became an annual occurrence, and every program director seemed to agree that it was enormously valuable. One of the recommendations stemming from the first conference was authorization for the explicit cooperation between and among Regional Medical Programs. Whether or not that turned out to be a key official factor in the pattern, it seems clear that there was fairly extensive communication among RMPs and especially their executive directors. The RMP directors group also proved to be a fertile source of leadership for other health policy and administrative positions. Stanley Olson came from the Tennessee Mid-South Program to be director of RMP. The guiding spirit of the Missouri RMP, Vernon Wilson, came to Washington in 1971 to be Administrator of the Health Services and Mental Health Administration, working closely with Monty Duval, the new (1971) Assistant Secretary for Health and the guiding spirit of the Arizona RMP. Both these distinguished physicians and medical school deans were selected with the active participation of Elliot Richardson, who would become Secretary of Health, Education and Welfare in June of 1970.

The formal authority of the Association of Regional Medical Programs was not tested until later. The informal grapevine had been working strongly from the beginning, and became particularly active upon hearing some stunning news contained in President Nixon's proposed budget for FY 1974.

In January 1973 Elliot Richardson left HEW to become Attorney General. The new HEW Secretary was Casper Weinberger, recently director of the Office of Management and Budget. Almost simultaneous with that change, the President wrote off Regional Medical Programs by not asking for any funds for their continuance in his budget for the 1974 fiscal year. Not that presidential action would necessarily be accepted. The Congress remained in Democratic hands and the House Interstate and Foreign Commerce Committee and its Health subcommittee had, after all, been the official parents of Regional Medical Programs. It was in that committee that the actual language — including "regional cooperative arrangements" -- was formulated and ultimately became law.

Paul Rogers, Chairman on the Subcommittee on Public Health and Environment, asked the administration to come and explain to the committee why, only a short time after the Department of Health, Education and Welfare representatives had praised the program and why, since no new programs were offered to replace the role of RMPs in communities, it proposed to eliminate them. [1] Carrying the burden of the argument of the administration was Dr. John Zapp, D.D.S., Deputy Assistant Secretary for Legislation. He brought with him Dr. Harold Margulies, who had been Director of the RMP Service for two years. It was, Dr. Zapp indicated, a dual reason. In the first place, the President had determined that the "administration's budget would not exceed reasonable projections of federal funding ability without increased taxation." [2] Second, from the outset, "Regional Medical Programs has had great difficulty defining a clear role for itself in concentrating its efforts and resources on a few, well-selected target areas." [3] Dr. Zapp asserted that more than one half billion dollars had been expended in RMPs since their creation, and there was very little to show for it.

Not that the President was indifferent to the federal government's role in health. Indeed, the administration wanted to give first priority to reducing financial barriers that limited access to care. [4] Soon, said Dr. Zapp, the President would be submitting a national health insurance plan to Congress and meanwhile his administration would continue to rely on existing major programs -- presumably including Medicare, Medicaid, the National Institutes of Health, the Food and Drug Administration. Otherwise "a more limited federal role and increased reliance of the capabilities of local and private sectors are indicated...." [5]

So Regional Medical Programs had to go. Beyond their not having accomplished anything of coherence and significance, Zapp asserted that they were spending 40% of their funds on administration and overhead. Not only that, but federal funds were paying for 1,400 salaried officials around the country. [6]

> There is no significant evidence that RMPs have achieved their goal of getting research advances into regular, large-scale practice. The training programs undertaken are typically of limited scope and duration, and there is no substantiating evidence that these have had a significant impact on actual medical practice or in demonstrating improved quality care. [7]

What the administration proposed was to continue certain activities, particularly those in demonstration and heart disease, cancer, and kidney disease through programs of the National Institutes of Health. With respect to planning, it should be the Comprehensive Health Planning Program that took over some of the responsibilities of RMP. Indeed, the CRMP-CHP overlap was another reason for getting rid of RMPs. "It is difficult to have a CHP agency with responsibility for the health planning for an area while another federally supported program, an RMP, is implementing activities in that same area based on its own planning and priority settings... Given the narrower provider base of RMP, this is not always consistent with broader community and consumer health needs and interests." [8]

The administration was not arguing, said Dr. Zapp, that "Regional Medical Programs had no achievements and accomplishments." [9] There were in fact several, the first being that they had "fostered development of a local decision making and implementing mechanism that constitutes a framework for a broad spectrum of provider interest, institutions and groups to cooperatively address problems." [10] And that, he added, should be helpful to new Professional Standards Review endeavors.

RMPs had also "served as a modest force for institutional reform in the health arena". They may have helped, for example, to reduce in some regions the gap between the research/educational focus of medical schools and the patient service needs of community hospitals and practicing physicians. They definitely had "contributed to the launching of other federal health initiatives." [11] These included the Emergency Medical Service Programs, recently adopted as a separate national program by the federal government. And not to worry: RMPs had already found continuation support "albeit usually at a reduced level, for about one half of the operational projects initiated with RMP grants." [12] In summary, Regional Medical Programs have not achieved the promise they held, according to Dr. Zapp. He asserted that "in our considered judgment, its accomplishments have not been commensurate with the costs," which totalled more than $500 million. [13]

The House hearings which took place in early May 1973 were a recapitulation of the history, and the diversity, of Regional Medical Programs. But the men who served on the committee, beginning with the Chairman, Paul Rogers of Florida, would not simply accept what the administration recommended. Indeed, Paul Rogers had established himself as an independent voice when he tried valiantly, though ultimately unsuccessfully, to stave off the Nixon-Kennedy bill to create a new cancer authority and remove the Cancer Institute from direct NIH control. [14] He was, by this time, broadly and deeply familiar with all aspects of health care and the federal programs dealing with them. He was a good lawyer and he was a good chairman. Neither he nor his colleagues on the committee were going to permit the administration easily to terminate RMPs.

Dr. Tim Lee Carter, the ranking Republican on the committee, who eight years earlier had been persuaded by Dr. DeBakey that Regional Medical Programs were a good thing, seemed a little bit unhappy with the President's proposal to terminate them, although he manifested some unhappiness with the program itself, asserting that it had not followed its original purpose of focusing on heart disease, cancer and stroke. [15] Congressman Richardson Preyer of North Carolina agreed that there probably was some unevenness of the quality of the programs across the country -- "I guess that is true for any program" -- but he knew for certain, from direct experience, that the North Carolina Regional Medical Program was a good one. [16]

Rep. Bill Roy, the Democrat and physician from Kansas, was

astounded that the administration's view of RMP could change so dramatically so fast. He grilled Dr. Margolies in particular:

> Mr. Roy: Is it true that you, Dr. Margolies, said in January 1972 that RMP was the best of all federal programs? Is that a proper phrasing of what you said?
>
> Dr. Margolies: It is possible that is what I said.
>
> Mr. Roy: What happened between January of `72 and January of `73.
>
> Dr. Margolies: Let me go back and give as candid an answer as I can. Before I joined Regional Medical Programs, I had great doubts about it. I thought it was a so-so program, and my interest was modest.
>
> When I became director of the program it was in great trouble, but I entered it enthusiastically. I pursued it as vigorously as I could. I could not have been in it and remained objective about it, and when I worked for it, I worked for it with all my heart. When I said warm things about it, it was partly because I wanted to transfer my enthusiasm and support to what is really a remarkable group of people, the coordinators of RMPs. [17]

What had also happened was that Dr. Margolies had now been enlisted by his superiors in the Department in Health, Education and Welfare to help reorder federal health policies and priorities. So, "placing the program in the total context and with the range of issues Dr. Zapp has laid out, I have had to be more objective, more withdrawn, and take a view within a larger setting." [18] As to what had happened specifically in the last year: "Nothing remarkable happened as I had to look at this program in what I think is much wiser frame of reference with a total look at the health delivery system and a more cautious use of funds to get the job done." [19]

Congressman James Hastings (Republican, New York) had also been on the committee when the original legislation was enacted, and he had kept up with the Regional Medical Program his part of the State and perhaps more generally. He proposed a compromise: "Why not continue Regional Medical Program for a year while both the executive and legislative branches have more careful evaluations of their value, the overlap between RMP and other programs, possible sources of continuation of the best programs?"

Being a good Republican as well as a good member of the

committee, and probably being as uncomfortable in defending RMPs as Dr. Zapp and Margolies were in urging their disembowelment, Congressman Hastings said: "I do not think we are that far apart. I would once again plead with you that we have the opportunity to discuss that type of question before not just the subcommittee but all interested parties throughout this country, who are in fact interested in improving our health delivery system and I think that is what we are talking about." [20]

The grilling continued. Had Regional Medical Program services done their own assessment of the RMPs across the country? Yes, according to the criteria in three areas: performance, process and substantive proposed programs, the criteria specified in four pages of detail. Would Mr. Margolies provide the most recent ratings, those of January 1973? He did so. [21] In fact, Chairman Rogers already had the ratings at hand. He reported to his colleagues, in the presence of Dr. Zapp and Dr. Margolies, that "out of 56 only 14 were rated as less than good, the others good or excellent." [22] So the question to the administration officials was: "What did you use as a basis for saying the programs should be phased out after this appraisal on January 31, 1973? That was just a few months ago." [23]

As is typical of congressional oversight hearings, and especially true in the case of those organized by legislative masters like Congressman Rogers, the hearings proceeded from the administration witnesses to those who took other points of view. These included Dr. William J. Hagood, speaking for the Virginia Medical Society and the American Academy Family Practice who strongly urged a one-year extension. He did not wish, he said, "to portray a picture devoid of problems and frustrations." Indeed, "being involved in RMP has been one of the most frustrating exercises with which I've ever been associated. The reason for this is the very reason I am before you today. It is, for the lack of a better term, the fickleness of the federal government." [24]

> We have had our funding levels shifted, funds taken away without notice, promises broken, commitments unmet, told one thing one day and another thing another day, and our credibility compromised because of the arbitrary and capricious behavior of federal bureaucrats more interested in form than substance.[25]

Similar sentiments are expressed by Dr. Robert Carter, the Dean of the University of Minnesota Medical School. [26]

A panel of Regional Medical Program coordinators testified. These included Dr. John R.F. Ingall, Executive Director of the Lakes Area RMP; Dr. H. Philip Hampton, Chairman of the Board of the Florida Regional Medical Program; Dr. William McBeath, Director of the Ohio Valley Regional Medical Program; which included Kentucky; and Paul D. Ward, Executive Director of the California Committee on Regional Medical Programs. All testified to the difficulty of operating Regional Medical Programs as enterprises intended to be local in organization and direction and democratic in-process, in the context of changing federal directives.

Dr. Bill McBeath's presence was almost certainly designed to reassure the ranking Republican on the committee, Dr. Carter of Kentucky. He directed the Ohio Valley Regional Medical Program which encompassed much of Kentucky, including the university medical centers at Lexington and Louisville as well as that in Cincinnati. In fact, it was one of the more interesting programs in its delineation, for it served an area covering 141 counties in four states with a total population of six million people. Dr. McBeath described a variety of programs including a number in Kentucky, but unfortunately none of those he mentioned -- given the Nixon administration's preferences and emphases -- had the words "heart disease," "cancer," or "stroke" in them. Dr. Carter had apparently not favored the more general direction: "I still say that you are differing from the intent of the legislation, in that it should be focused on heart and cancer, stroke and kidney." [27]

Dr. McBeath regretted that Congressman Carter had not found among the list of programs about Kentucky projects "how the people in your district have been served." Dr. Carter responded with his typical candor: "I may have gotten a catalogue or something from you, but no information that is meaningful. If you want to get information to your representative, write on one or two sheets of paper and no more because he has no time for catalogues." [28] Dr. Ingall's congressman, James Hastings, was more amenable to his constituents' responses, and he again expressed the hope that the program would be extended for a year.

Paul Ward specified the reason the original disease categories were no longer exclusively followed. That was because, in February 1970, Secretary of Health Education and Welfare Robert Finch, in his White Paper on the new administration's health priorities, emphasized that RMPs should join other agencies in developing "the creation of primary care for those people that did not have it. These included Indians, migrant workers, and poor people in the inner city." In response, said Mr. Ward, a group of coordinators had a long meeting with the Secretary and his colleagues and "came to a general agreement on how the program should proceed along the Finch priorities." [29]

Bill Roy summed up the impression of most members of the committee and most people involved in Regional Medical Programs. The Nixon administration had urged decategorization and an emphasis on primary care; the Regional Medical Programs had been good enough to comply, and now the program was being terminated because it had lost its focus, had "never carved out a role for itself." [30] That was too disingenuous, too hypocritical.

The Congress continued the program for another year. The vote in favor was overwhelming: in the Senate, 94 to zero; in the House, 372 to one.

Notes:

1. U.S. House of Representatives, Committee on Interstates and Foreign Commerce, "Oversight Hearings on Regional Medical Programs," May 8, 1973. p.1.
2. Ibid., p.2
3. Ibid., p.3
4. Ibid.
5. Ibid.
6. Ibid., p.4
7. Ibid.
8. Ibid.
9. Ibid., p. 5
10. Ibid.
11. Ibid.
12. Ibid., p.6
13. Ibid.
14. See Stephen P. Strickland, Politics, Science and Dread Disease (Cambridge, Mass: Harvard University Press, 1972), Chapter XII, esp. pp. 280-287
15. Oversight hearings, May 1973, op.cit., pp.8-14, p.20
16. Ibid., p.7
17. Ibid., p.14

18. Ibid.
19. Ibid.
20. Ibid., pp.22,23
21. Ibid., pp-23-30
22. Ibid., p.141
23. Ibid.
24. Ibid., p.166
25. Ibid.
26. Ibid., pp.168-170
27. Ibid., p.237
28. Ibid.
29. Ibid., p.244
30. Ibid., pp.244-245

Chapter 14

Demise and Legacy

Congress extended the RMP authority in 1973, and voted the program appropriations for the next year. But the funds were promptly impounded by the administration. Friends of the Regional Medical Programs, especially the program executive directors and some members of their Regional Advisory groups, were appalled. They had already suspected the administration of insincerity and capriciousness. Now they were convinced of its perfidy. The Association of Regional Medical Programs filed suit in federal court, charging violation of the law, and won. Secretary Weinberger had no choice but to release the $218 million in question, even though he profoundly regretted such funds — on top of the half a billion dollars expended on RMPs since the beginning -- "being directed into this dubious direction."[1]

It seemed clear to Paul Ward of California that the main reason for the Secretary's opposition to RMPs was philosophical. The two men had battled on many past occasions in California, over policy, government's role, and budgetary issues. Backed by his colleagues across the country, Mr. Ward had launched the first successful counterattack, the law suit. The war continued in the halls of Congress, in deliberations of health associations, and on the editorial pages of medical journals.

In the eyes of the proximate policy makers -- those in the Congress and the subordinate agencies of HEW -- the legal victory was merely a stay of execution. Some of the program directors knew that the country would not come to their rescue. One of the problems, said Jim Haviland of the University of Washington, was that RMPs had done such an effective job as initiators and facilitators that most people in a community who were benefitting from an RMP program did not know where the idea or the money came from. Not a single congressman went out and ran for re-election, in 1974, on the grounds that if returned to office, he or she would ensure the continuance of Regional Medical Programs. Dr. John Packard in Alabama later identified as a key failure of his program that of not paying enough attention to public relations. Other RMP directors echoed the sentiments. Even Paul Rogers, one of the authors and staunch friends of RMP, did not believe the cause was so supremely important that he and his committee colleagues should again don armor and wage a new fight.

In fact, none of the distinctive constituencies of RMP seemed to feel sufficiently strongly that they wanted to get into another fray. Some were advancing their particular interests in other ways. The American Cancer Society and the American Heart Association had won great victories in enlarging the authorities of their favorite NIH institutes, including those for demonstration projects, under the National Cancer Act of 1971 and the National Heart, Lung and Blood Institute Act of 1972.

Medical schools increasingly had other federal sources of support. And even medical schools which had been at the center of RMPs had long since recognized that the original hope for gradually but steadily increasing sums of money for the national program and for their institutions was turning into fantasy. Case-Western Reserve was apparently one such institution. In 1992, nobody who had been in a leadership position at the Medical School in RMP days could remember much about the program. John Thompson of Yale said: "The schools just got tired of all that RMP stuff."

Meanwhile, state departments of health were delighted with the prospect of increased support and increased funds. They had always viewed RMPs with concern. After all, what had been created in the Heart Disease, Cancer and Stroke Amendments of 1965 was a network of new organizations not under the control of state, county or other health departments but extending across traditional jurisdictional boundaries. Not only that, but RMPs involved health care professionals and lay persons in decisions about health care resources and systems. It was this concern which, soon after the passage of RMP, prompted the Johnson administration and the Congress to "redress the balance," and strengthen state and local planning officials' status with authority for health systems agencies. State health officials had applauded Nixon administration proposals, first offered in 1973 and reintroduced a year later, to merge some of the functions of Regional Medical Programs and Health Systems Agencies and give the planning agencies the lead.

There was general agreement, in 1974, that the rise in federal expenditures for health -- from $4 billion in fiscal 1965 to $26 billion in 1975 -- was in itself a reason to slow down and, if possible, cut back. This agreement, however, simply set off even more strenuous struggles among different interests about what to do about it. Each group, whether that still pushing for increases in the NIH budget or another which thought federal support for HMOs should move at a faster pace, pushed budgetary priorities in sharply different, sometimes directly opposite, directions.

Still, even those who from a state or local RMP perspective saw what the overall problem was, deeply resented the reasons offered by the administration for the planned execution. Secretary Weinberger repeated precisely, almost word for word, in August 1974, the testimony John Zapp gave before Congress in May 1973: "From the outset the RMP has had great difficulty in defining a clear role for itself in concentrating its efforts and resources on even a few, well-selected target areas. At the same time, it has been unsuccessful in reconciling the conflicting and changing emphases between categorical disease activities and comprehensive health problems."[2] He denied that RMPs had in any significant way "produced the regionalized systems of health care originally envisioned at the program's outset." And finally: "It is difficult to have a comprehensive health planning agency with the responsibility with the health planning for an area while in other federally-supported program and RMP is implementing activities in that same area based on its own planning and priorities."[3]

So the word went out, from the Acting Director's Office of RMP, that individual programs must plan their orderly termination, with no funds to be expended after June 30, 1975. Adding vinegar to the already bitter wine, simultaneous directives ordered the programs to spend millions of dollars on kidney disease and diabetes programs. Thus the directors of Regional Medical Programs, and their advisory groups, went about the business of closing down shop. Some were philosophical, some were bitter, all were dutiful. Of the remaining business, the most important was to try to secure support for the continuance of the best

RMP projects from other sources. This happened in a very significant number of cases. The State of Missouri took over the RMP kidney dialysis program. The State of Maryland adopted the blood bank program created, as one of its best products, by the Maryland RMP.

The next task, undertaken by many of the programs, was a self-appointed one. It was to record the consequences of their respective Regional Medical Programs over the decade of their formal existence. Already, the directors had together, under Paul Ward's aegis, summed up "progress and assessment of impact" in the course of the last legislative debate in mid-1973.[4] Their report asserted that the number of people directly served by RMPs across the country in that year alone totalled almost 14 million. Of these, 5.7 million were identified as having received primary care; over four million received the benefits of emergency medical services and approximately 1.5 million patients with heart disease, cancer and stroke received care.[5] Over 100,000 Americans, according to the report, were served by health providers to whom RMP had given new or improved skills. In 1973 alone, the programs claimed to have provided training for more than 150,000 professionals. Meanwhile, to make the system work, some 19,000 regular volunteers had contributed time and energy to RMPs, "often at considerable personal financial sacrifice, to study and act upon health problems in a way that is best suited to local situations."[6] Furthermore, of this number, "over 2,600 advisors are from a minority population which represents a significant proportion compared to national averages."[7]

According to the report, the approximately $117 million spent through RMPs in 1973 represented the following functional contributions: $31 million for more effective use of manpower; $37 million to improve accessibility and availability of primary medical care, including emergency care; $26.6 million to support regionalization of secondary and tertiary care, including care of heart, cancer, stroke and kidney patients; $14.6 million on efforts to assure appropriate quality of care; and only $7.5 million on administrative costs.[8] The latter figure, according to Mr. Ward, amounted to about 7 percent of the total cost of the program -- not the 20 percent claimed by the Administration.[9]

Thirty years later, reviews of final reports of the Regional Medical Programs and appraisals from other sources suggest both enormous diversity in overall reach, and a consistent, central core of programs which accorded both with the original purposes of the program and its gradually expanded authority. Among the more unusual legacies was the support of new medical schools. The Missouri Regional Medical Program assisted in the development of a two-year medical school in Kansas City. Two RMPs in Los Angeles helped created the Charles R. Drew Graduate Medical School there. In the case of the Mountain States, an RMP grant to the Western Interstate Commission of Higher Education was the building block on which the University of Nevada Medical School began.

The use of computers and related technologies in diagnosis and monitoring treatment, pioneered in Missouri and several other places in the late 1960's, has now become standard across the country. Health education centers, such as those still operating in North Carolina, Washington, and in many other places as well, sometimes had their organizational origins in RMP grants and in every case were supported by a Regional Medical Program. RMP consistently supported the development of medical libraries and the National Medical Library System, even though there was, throughout its history, separate national authority for such support. Regarding medical communications, one review stated that the dial access libraries in medical schools throughout various states "were established under RMP sponsorship or system."

Consistent, large activities were training programs for physicians, nurses and other health professionals in emergency medical services and in coronary intensive care units. Every RMP made a major investment in these two areas. Many of the first coronary intensive care units and E.M.S. programs were begun with RMP funds. Most continue today all across the country. This sustained effort has surely contributed to the significant decrease in death by heart attack in the last thirty years.

In the last year, 1975, the larger regional programs were supporting scores of projects covering a wide array of subjects and needs. The Missouri RMP, for example, operated 77 projects in fiscal year 1974-75, which amounted to approximately half those it had undertaken in the decade. In this national array, there were clearly some activities that were unusual along with many that were not; some were pioneering, others were traditional or derivative. Naturally, program results also varied considerably. By most accounts, including those registered thirty years ago and those collected in the 1990s, the aggregate impact of the program was significant and beneficial.

At the behest of the national office, Regional Medical Programs from an early date constructed elaborate evaluation criteria. But measurements of success, or lack of it, in such enterprises remain elusive. The enthusiasm of the former executive directors of Regional Medical Programs, of the key staff, and members of the advisory groups is remarkably -- although not perfectly -- consistent. The great majority remember the program fondly and positively. A few think such enthusiasm is unwarranted.

Both the praising and the occasional negative assessments come from different levels. One physician attending the December 1991 conference on Regional Medical Programs at the National Library of Medicine reported feeling a little incredulous at the praise heaped on RMPs by those who had been involved in its national direction or its local programs. The large metropolitan area RMP he knew -- that encompassing the Nation's Capital — had not been, by anyone's account, a particularly good one. Beyond that, he mused, perhaps his reaction stemmed from the fact that his role in RMP was at a lower level than those reporting: "I felt like a private at a reunion of generals."

Nonetheless, if the positive assessments are not universal, they are certainly dominant. And there is consensus that one contribution stands above all the rest. It is that RMPs inspired more productive conversations and cooperative ventures among health care providers and educators, officials and lay citizens, some of which last to this day, than any other source or force. That legacy may become newly relevant and valuable when the next health crisis in America occurs -- or is proclaimed. For it is only crises that seem to move the nation and its leaders to concerted action, to forge new policies that are commensurate with the need.

Some health crises are not predictable. Some are. That which is looming as a new century begins stems from the same dilemma which inspired President Johnson to launch his multiple plans in the 1960s and President Clinton to try to launch his grand plan in 1993: Too many Americans in too many circumstances remain outside the circle of medical care.

Focused dialogue leading to collaborative action on real problems is what Regional Medical Programs represented. That approach can work again, on the regional, state and national level. In an ideal world it could work even now, before the new crisis is discovered and declared.

Notes:

1. Casper W. Weinberger, "The Guideposts in the RMP Odessey," Western Medical Journal, Aug. 1974, p. 159.
2. Ibid.
3. Ibid.
4. "Special Progress Report: Regional Medical Programs, included in "Regional Medical Programs - oversight Hearings," House Committee on Interstate and Foreign Commerce, Subcommittee on Public Health and Environment. 93rd Congress, First Session. May 8, 1973, pp. 221-232.
5. Ibid., Tables I and II, P. 222.
6. Ibid., P. 226.
7. Ibid., p. 227
8. Ibid., Table VII, p. 228.
9. "Oversight Hearings," May 8, 1973, op. cit., p. 220.

INDEX

134

Jacksonville (Fla) 65
James, George 43
Johnson, Lyndon B. (LBJ) 1-4, 10, 13,
   19, 21, 26, 29, 37, 39, 47, 52, 79-80,
   84-85, 131
Johnson Administration, 104, 108,
   110, 127

Kansas, University Medical Center
   81
Kansas Medical Society 81-82
Kansas RMP, 81
Kellogg Foundation, 97
Kennedy, Edward (Ted), 115
Kennedy, John F., 2, 37
Kimmel, Bill, 82
King, Martin Luther, Jr. General
Hospital, 105
King, Rep. , 18
King, Dr. Kenton, 80
Kirksville (Mo) 81
Kissick, William 6, 33
Klapper, Margaret 73-75
Knowles, John, 86

Lakes Area RMP, 123
Lasker, Albert, 3, 4, 5, 29
Lasker, Mary, 2, 3, 5, 6, 29, 34, 115
Las Vegas, 103
Lee, Philip R., 20
Lein, Jack, 93, 95
Lewis, Charles, 81
Lilienfeld, Abraham, 5
Lindberg, Donald A. B., 82-83, 86-88
Loma Linda University Medical
School, 101, 103
Long Island (NY), 41
Los Angeles County Medical
Association, 17, 100
Louisville Courier Journal, 5

Macon (Ga), 60
MacArthur, Douglas, 102
Magnuson, Warren, 93
Mahoney, Florence, 34, 41
Maine, 32
Malden, John, 60

Margulies, Harold, 111, 118, 121-122
Marston, Robert Q., 25, 27, 100, 117
Maryland RMP, 129
Massachusettes, 32
Massachusettes General Hospital, 86
Mayer, Eugene,
Mayer, William D., 26, 60
McBeath, William, 123
McDonald, Ian 17, 18
McLaughlin, Mary, 43
Meador, Cliff, 73
Medicaid, 1, 4, 6, 19, 23, 87, 119
Medical Information Service in
   Telephone (MIST), 73-76
Medicare, 1,4, 6, 19, 23, 87, 110, 119
Medic One, 98
Medlars, 10, 104
Meyer, John, 5
Miami (Fla), 65
Michigan RMP, 114
Minnesota, University of,
Minority populations (health
   problems) 98, 105
Mississippi, University of, 25
Mississippi River, 33, 68, 81
Missouri, Cancer Society, 80, 82;
   Farm Bureau, 89; Federation of
   Women's Clerks, 89; Heart
   Association, 80, 82; Hospital
   Assoc., 82; Kidney Foundation, 82;
   Kidney Program, 83; Nursing Home
   Assoc., 82; Regional Advisory
   Group, 84; RMP, 78-91, 117, 130;
   School of Journalism, 83; School of
   Medicine, 26, 78-79; School of
   Nursing, 82; State Health
   Department, 79; State Medical
   Association, 80-84
Mobile (Ala), 71
Modern Medicine, 17
Montana, 92, 94
Montgomery (Ala), 71
Mountain, Joseph, 34
Mountain Report, 35
Moyer, William, 82
Musser, Marc J., 52

Nassau County (NY), 41